High Altitude
Illness and Wellness

by Charles Houston

ICS BOOKS, Inc.
Merrillville, Indiana

HIGH ALTITUDE: Illness and Wellness
Copyright © 1993 Charles S. Houston

10 9 8 7 6 5 4 3 2 1

Printed in U.S.A.

Published by:
ICS Books, Inc.
1370 E. 86th Place
Merrillville, IN 46410
800-541-7323

Library of Congress Cataloging-in-Publication Data

Houston, Charles S.
    High Altitude : illness and wellness / by Charles Houston.
       p.   cm.
    Includes index.
    ISBN 0-934802-72-6 : $6.99
    1. Altitude, Influence of. 2. Acclimatization   I. Title.
QP82.2.A4H68 1993
616.9'893--dc20   **92-47107**
                                              CIP

TABLE OF CONTENTS

FURTHER READING

INTRODUCTION: WHAT'S IT ALL ABOUT? i

1. THE ATMOSPHERE AROUND US 1

2. A FEELING FOR MOUNTAINS 7

3. GOING HIGHER 11

4. MOVING AIR: VENTILATION 15

5. MOVING BLOOD: CIRCULATION 23

6. THE VITAL FLUID 29

7. CELLS: THE ULTIMATE USERS 39

8. MOUNTAIN SICKNESS 43

9. STAYING WELL AT ALTITUDE 63

INDEX 70

FURTHER READING

HIGH ALTITUDE, PHYSIOLOGY
Edited by John B. West
Van Nostrand Reinhold. 1981

THE MONTGOLFIER BROTHERS
AND THE INVENTIONS OF AVIATION, 1783-1784
Charles S. Gillespie
Princeton University Press. 1983

GOING HIGHER: THE STORY OF MAN AND ALTITUDE
Charles S. Houston
Little, Brown and Company. 1987.

HIGH ALTITUDE MEDICINE AND PHYSIOLOGY
Michael P. Ward, James S. Milledge and John B. West
University of Pennsylvania Press. 1989

INTRODUCTION: WHAT'S THIS ALL ABOUT?

On September 2, 1891, a young French physician lay desperately ill high on Mont Blanc. He had hurried up from the village of Chamonix to help build a new observatory. The next day he climbed to the summit (4,800 meters; 15,771 feet), and within twenty-four hours wrote to his brother that, due to mountain sickness, he had never passed so terrible a night. He died three days after arrival, a victim of altitude, and was called "a martyr to science." His is the first well-documented case of high altitude pulmonary edema.

Others experienced mountain sickness even longer ago. The huge *History of the Han Dynasty,* written by Ban Gu a few decades into the Christian era, contains a dramatic warning written to Emperor Wudi by one of his generals:

> South of Mount Pishan [in the Karakoram range] the travellers have to climb over Mount Greater Headache, Mount Lesser Headache, and the Fever Hill, where they will develop a fever, turn pallid, feel a headache, and vomit, which also occurs in asses and other animals without exception. Then there are the Three Pools and the Rocky Hill, where the path narrows down to a width of one and a half feet in some places and stretches for thirty li. Trudging beside the fathomless abysses, the travellers and their animals have to support each other with ropes. On this journey of more than 2000 li to Hondu, animals will be dashed to pieces before they fall halfway into a deep gorge, while human bodies will never be recovered. Dangers and casualties are too numerous to count.

In the 1400s, while campaigning on the high plateau of Central Asia, a Moslem warlord named Mirza Muhammad Haider described a strange affliction called "dam-giri" that killed many of his men and horses.

By the start of the twentieth century the cause of the several forms of mountain sickness had been recognized and both prevention and treatment were known. Nevertheless, as I write, a young British pilot has just died from altitude illness while searching for a wrecked aircraft in the Himalayan foothills. As an experienced and well-trained pilot he should have known about the dangers of altitude.

Each year around the world hundreds of young, strong, healthy people— soldiers, trekkers, climbers, and ordinary tourists—die from avoidable altitude illness. Hundreds of thousands become ill because they do not know, or choose to ignore, how dependent we humans are on an adequate and uninterrupted supply of oxygen.

The story of how we came to know something of the physical universe around us and the physiological universe within our bodies is a fascinating one, taking us from ignorance and superstition to a glimmering understanding life. We have learned through trial and error, death and disappointment, and from the work of our predecessors. Truly, "even pygmies, standing on the shoulders of giants, can see more than the giants themselves."

In this small book I will describe briefly but respectfully what the pioneers did and concluded and how we have come to where we are today (chapters 1 to 3). Some of them were wrong of course, and led us astray. However, even their mistakes illuminate the future, and who knows but that some mistaken paths may someday be useful by-ways.

To help the reader understand wellness and sickness at altitude, I will describe how we obtain and use oxygen and how essential it is to life (chapters 4 to 7). I have described how and why we breathe and why and how the heart pumps blood throughout the body. It is important to understand how hemoglobin works and to be familiar with a few of the laws of physics that control these functions. I've also taken a quick look at that complicated factory—the living cell. There is a little sophisticated science here which I hope will satisfy the scientists, but basically this book is for the nontechnical reader.

On this foundation I will describe the problems that confront us as we climb toward the sky, commonly known as mountain sickness (chapter 8), and the adaptations that enable us, and even more amazingly some animals, to survive on high, that is, the process of acclimatization (chapter 9).

"Altitude" means different things to different people. I think of 2,400 to 3,600 meters (8,000 to 12,000 feet) as moderate altitude, 4,500 to 5,400 meters (15,000 to 18,000 feet) as high altitude, and over 6,600 meters (22,000 feet) as very high or extreme altitude. Most of this book, like most research in the past, describes what happens at moderate altitude, and this is what I mean when I simply write *altitude* without a qualifier. I hope you will keep in mind that even moderate altitude can be dangerous: tragedies and mistakes can occur, and have occurred, as low as 2,400 meters. Make no mistake: altitude, like lack of oxygen anywhere, can cripple or kill. As Joseph Barcroft wrote, "Hypoxia halts the works and wrecks the machinery."

Many medical texts explain breathing, circulation, and the functions of blood in great detail. Thousands of articles have been written about lack of oxygen and about altitude. Hundreds of thousands of skiers, hikers, climbers and tourists are experiencing the effects of high altitude every day. My 1987 book, *Going Higher: The Story of Man and Altitude,* has an extensive bibliography, and others are also available. Why write yet another book about altitude sickness?

First of all, I am fascinated by history and by our predecessors, so many of whom are "unwept, unhonored, and unsung," although they laid the corner stones of what we know today. I love to dig up treasures of the musty past to show to others. More importantly, however, I am dedicated to telling people about how their bodies work, how they can stay well, and why they may get sick if or when they lack oxygen. Almost everyone is interested in his or her body and often curious about the whys and hows of its function or malfunction. In addition, there are many misconceptions about how the human body works, and even that which is correct is often hard to understand. Here I have tried to write in ordinary language, not in medical jargon.

Mountains tug at the spirit and the heart. As a long-time mountaineer I've been there, learned that. As a practicing doctor I've seen what happens when people don't have enough of this "vital spirit," oxygen, either on mountains or in the sick room. The healthy man or woman climbing high in the Himalayas has much in common with the frail patient panting in bed because of emphysema or pneumonia. We need to learn more about these similarities.

Finally, there's all the rest of life on Earth. How can birds go so much higher than we can? How do bears and woodchucks sleep, barely breathing, during long winter months? How can whales and seals stay under water ten or twenty times as long as we can? How do insects breathe? How does the chick embryo get oxygen in its egg? I can't answer these questions in this small book, but I hope my readers will ask them and think about them, and perhaps some will visit these tempting, only partially explored areas.

This book's ostensible purpose is to explain why you may get sick if you go into the mountains imprudently, and how you can stay well. Some readers' lives may be saved by this information. That's the best part of medicine—prevention.

But there's more. We are put together in a wondrous way. We are more intricate than the wildest fancy can conceive. Though other organisms have some mechanisms much like ours, we alone are able to examine, analyze, and explain at least in part how our bodies work. I've tried to express some of the wonder we should feel when we look at all life, but especially our own.

Charles S. Houston, MD
Burlington Vermont
November 17, 1992

1. THE ATMOSPHERE AROUND US

Picture a miner, thousands of years ago, deep underground. He learned that when his torch flickered and went out, he would become sick and might even die. That pioneer could not associate his sickness with the air he breathed because the concept of air had not evolved. Yet all unwittingly, he made the first connection between air, combustion, and life.

Many centuries later philosophers speculated about the invisible, impalpable substance in which they lived. Aristotle wrote that ". . . every body has weight, except fire, even air. It is proof that an inflated bladder weighs more than an empty one." Yet even he could not believe that space could be empty, and he could not accept the fact that a vacuum could exist.

People slowly came to recognize the process of breathing, the apparatus that moves air in and out of the body, and the dependence of life on breathing. The heart, blood, and lungs were described, though many centuries would pass before their interactions were defined. Even the physical properties of air were not appreciated until 1618 when a daring young student named Isaac Beeckman wrote, "It happens that air, in the manner of water, presses upon things and compresses them." He came into immediate conflict with the leading scientists of the day, who denied that air had weight and would not accept the possibility of a vacuum. Two decades later another youngster, Roman mathematician Gaspar Berti, serendipitously made a primitive barometer. He proved that a vacuum could exist and that air had weight. This discovery led Evangellista Torricelli to make the first mercury barometer.

In a famous experiment in 1654, Otto von Guericke evacuated the air from a globe consisting of two hemispheres pressed together. He dramatically

1

demonstrated the strength of air pressure when he showed that teams of horses could not separate the two hemispheres until the vacuum had been relieved. Beeckman and Berti were proven right!

A few years later Florin Périer took three Torricellian barometers to the top of a small mountain and showed that atmospheric pressure decreased with increasing altitude. The altimeter was born.

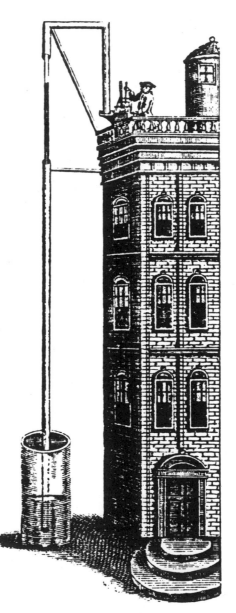

Figure 1-1

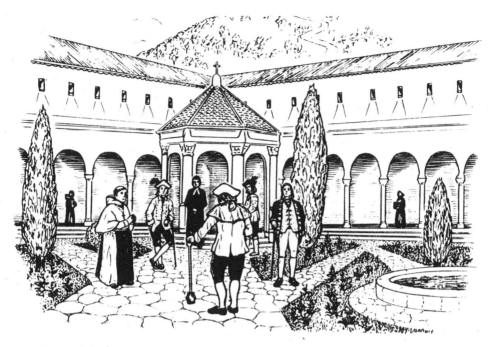

Figure 1-2

The Necessity of Air

Once air had been shown to have weight and to be compressible and removable from a sealed container, the next question was, "What is it made of?" von Guericke's vacuum pump provided means to study this mysterious substance, which could not be seen, felt, or smelled.

During this time, small groups of scholars were meeting in Britain and elsewhere to discuss the explosion of knowledge about the physical world triggered by the new instruments. They were insatiably curious, as their fascinating proceedings show. In 1662, after they had been meeting periodically for several years, one such group was formally granted a charter by the King of England and became the Royal Society of London, today one of the oldest scientific societies in the world.

Robert Boyle is perhaps the best known of this great group, but John Mayow was a better physiologist, and its curator, Robert Hooke, the busiest. Fellows of the young society hastened to use a modification of the Guericke pump to evacuate glass bell jars in which they observed what happened in a vacuum to lighted candles, mice, birds, and all manner of living organisms and inanimate objects. Very quickly they demonstrated what the ancient miners had observed: there is something in air that is necessary for life and for combustion. In a remarkably astute observation, John Mayow wrote:

"It is quite certain that animals in breathing draw from the air certain vital spirits. . . . That nitro-aerial spirit is by means of respiration transmitted into the mass of the blood and the fermentation and heating of the blood are produced by it."

The fellows of the Royal Society were immediately curious about the effects of a vacuum on humans, and Hooke proposed to make a device to accommodate a person. The fellows so ordered, and after some delay, on February 2, 1671, Hooke was seated in a large barrel from which the air was pumped by Boyle's modification of the Guericke device. Hooke was probably "taken up" only four thousand feet and felt no ill effects. Curiously, the published proceedings contain no further reference to this momentous adventure. It would be another hundred years before John Mayow's "vital spirit" was isolated.

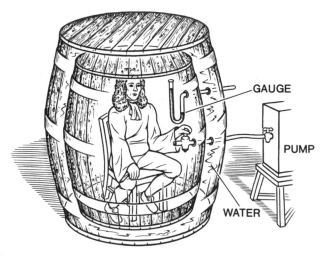

Figure 1-3

Robert Boyle "had taken notice of the unfitness for respiration [of the air], observed by the learned Acosta in the high mountains of Pariacaca" and questioned contemporary travellers about their experiences. One replied that the mountains "were exceeding high . . . and that whilst he was in the upper part of the mountain . . . he was reduced to fetch his breath much oftener than he was wont." Boyle was cautious enough not to exclude the possibility that "certain steams of a peculiar nature" might contribute to the sickness reported by these travellers. Nevertheless, he proposed that all air, wherever it came from, was the same, although it was thinner and lighter at altitude, and its composition was still a mystery.

The Gas Laws

Building on the work of Beeckman, Berti, Périer, Guericke, and others unremembered today, the great physical scientists Boyle, J.-A.-C. Charles, and John Dalton formulated the gas laws that define how gases behave when pressure or temperature are altered. These basic laws profoundly affect living processes and directly relate to our subject—altitude illness and wellness. Their formulation required one hundred and fifty years, and they are worth discussing.

Boyle's law (1662) states that the volume of a gas in an enclosed space varies inversely with the pressure on it; that is, when pressure increases, volume decreases (providing the temperature remains constant). Charles's law (1787) states that the volume of a gas increases as temperature increases (if pressure is kept constant). Dalton's law (1801) is more complicated: The total pressure of a mixture of gases is equal to the sum of the pressures of all the gases. In a closed space, the pressure of each gas is proportional to its percentage in the mixture. Each exerts the same pressure as it would if it were alone in the confined space. Dalton's law of partial pressure is fundamental to respiratory physiology.

The Composition of Air

The last piece of the puzzle of the atmosphere was determining the composition of this impalpable substance. Around 300 B.C. Erasistratus recognized that there was some relationship between the nature of life and the air we breath. He called this substance "pneuma" and anticipated John Mayow by calling one form of it a "vital spirit." Further identification languished for two thousand years.

In 1678 a prominent Danish physician named Olaus Borrichius (often known as Ole Borch), heated potassium nitrate and produced oxygen. He did not grasp the importance of this event, which went unremarked except perhaps by John Mayow. One hundred years later, in 1774, Carl Wilhelm Scheele, one of the great chemists of that century, sent a French colleague, Antoine-Laurent Lavoisier, a letter describing precisely how to isolate pure oxygen. Two years later Lavoisier and British clergyman William Priestley became famous when they simultaneously isolated oxygen. Scheele, however, remained torn between his strong belief in phlogiston and the contrary evidence of his experiments; his pioneering work, like that of Borch, has been virtually forgotten.

The phlogiston theory was advanced in 1669 by Johann Becher and is an example of belief supported by faith rather than observation. Becher and others postulated that substances were made of three kinds of earth: vitrifiable, mercurial, and combustible. When a substance was burned, Becher believed, the combustible portion was released. Georg Stahl named this portion "phlogiston" but disregarded the fact that the ash of a burned substance weighs less than the original. Some thought phlogiston might have a negative weight, others that it was a "principle" rather than a substance. The phlogiston theory stimulated many experiments and survived for more than a century, even for a short time after oxygen had been accepted by the scientific community.

In 1776 both Lavoisier and Priestley realized at once what they had found. Priestley opened a new door to physiology when he wrote:

"In this air as I had expected, a candle burned with a valid flame. In this air a mouse lived for a full half hour. . . . My reader will not wonder, that, having ascertained the superior goodness of dephlogisticated air by living mice . . . I should have the curiosity to taste it myself. . . . Who can tell but that, in time, this pure air may become a fashionable article in luxury.".

2. A FEELING FOR MOUNTAINS

Poets and travellers have long praised the beauty of great and sacred mountains. To the Christian world, the 121st Psalm is inspiring: "I will lift up mine eyes unto the hills from whence cometh mine help." Moses climbed a mountain to bring down the word of God. Isaiah urged, "Get thee up into the high mountains."

In the seventh century Li Bai, the Chinese poet-mountaineer wrote:

High above stands the loftiest peak
In the way of the God of the sun
Riding a chariot drawn by six dragons
Down below flows the winding stream
Foaming with impetuous waves
A barrier to the flying cranes
A headache to the climbing apes

Hundreds of minor and well-known poets have written and sung their admiration for mountains. A couplet from Byron's Childe Harold is a favorite:

I am not of myself but I become,
Portion of that around me, and to me
High mountains are a feeling
But the hum of busy cities torture.

Another of Byron's verses would be appropriate to our times:

Great things are done when men and mountains meet
That are not done by jostling in the street.

Mountains have always been a source of reverence, but until the nineteenth century mountains frightened rather than attracted most people. Doubtless some adventuresome hunters, and others looking for gems or minerals, were drawn to altitudes that might affect them, and hardy travellers might take the shortest way from one valley to another over a high pass. A few philosophers like Gessner or Petrarch went onto mountains for spiritual refreshment. It is not surprising that few ancient accounts of mountain sickness—or the perils of high altitude—have survived.

For most people big mountains were obstacles rather than destinations. Terrible storms could kill, and it was generally believed that dragons lived there. As Hobbes in 1651 said of the Middle Ages: "Men lived in . . . continual fear and danger of violent death; and the life of man [was] solitary, poor, nasty, brutish and short." Perhaps it is not surprising that they had neither time nor desire to climb mountains when they had crushing work to do at home. Or so we thought.

In 1988 two hikers crossing an Alpine glacier came across a body, huddled in a crevice between the ice and the rock wall, only recently exposed by unusually warm weather. The body, dressed in animal skins and carrying a crude alpenstock, a stone knife, and a copper axe, was quite well preserved. Evidently the man had bivouacked in a small depression and during the night, covered by a sudden fall of snow, had frozen to death. The glacier ice had preserved him almost perfectly. With great care the body was extricated, protected, and is being studied with all the skills of modern science. The conclusion: he had been high on the mountain, perhaps hunting, was familiar with mountain hazards and weather, carried a climbing aid and was dressed for the cold. He had lived and died some 5,300 years ago.

Early Explorers

But few adventurers, explorers, soldiers, or scientists seem to have attempted to climb and describe their experiences. Empedocles (490–430 B.C.), an amazingly versatile Greek philosopher-scientist, climbed Mount Etna, then higher than its present 3,271 meters (10,902 feet). According to legend, he leaped into the crater (some say to convince his followers of his divinity). The volcano spewed out his brass slippers but kept the philosopher. During his campaign against Athens, Philip of Macedon climbed Mount Haemus in the Balkans in 350 B.C., hoping to see both the Adriatic and the Aegean seas from the top; he could not.

In China Emperor Xuandi (91–49 B.C.) of the Han dynasty decreed that there were Five Sacred Mountains, each of which had some special attribute. They were said to be the abodes of celestial beings to which for generations sacrifices were made by emperors, prayers said by the people, and poems written by scholars.

During the third to sixth centuries monks travelled throughout Asia to spread Buddhism. Fa Hsien (A.D.334–420) wrote:

> The lakes in the Congling mountains are inhabited by poisonous dragons that breathe out poisonous clouds when enraged, causing downpours, blizzards and sandstorms from which no one can possibly escape alive. The Congling range is called "Snow Mountains" by the natives.

An outstanding early mountaineer was Xuan Zang (A.D.602–664), a Buddhist missionary, whose *Travels to the Western Regions* describes crossing passes and climbing mountains in the Tien Shan, Kun Lun, and Karakoram ranges. He really loved mountaineering; his highest climb was Lingshan (6,000 meters), making him the first high altitude climber and probably the earliest true mountaineer. He wrote:

> The journey is arduous and dangerous and the wind dreary and cold. Travellers are often attacked by fierce dragons so that they should neither wear red garments nor carry gourds with them, nor shout loudly. Even the slightest violation of these rules will invite disaster.

Marco Polo, journeying from Europe to China, said of the Pamir range:

> When the traveller leaves Wakhan he goes three days' journey toward the northeast, through mountains all the time, climbing so high that this is said to be the highest place in the world . . . fire is not so bright here nor of the same color as elsewhere, and food does not cook so well.

Then we find a real mountaineer, though the account of only one exploit seems to have survived: Peter II of Aragon (1174–1213) climbed Pic Canigou (2,740 meters; 9,135 feet) in the Pyrenees, simply to see what was on the summit. His report is reminiscent of Fa Hsien. He said there was a small lake on the summit from which a huge and horrible dragon emerged and flew about.

Like Peter of Aragon's Pic Canigou, Mount Pilatus (2,095 meters; 6,983 feet) in Switzerland was said to have a summit lake. Into this water legend had it that the body of Pontius Pilate was cast. If the lake were disturbed, terrible catastrophes were visited on the surrounding countryside. Today there is no lake on the summit!

Konrad Gessner is the first European writer whose description of love for mountains has survived. In his book *On the Admiration of Mountains* he wrote:

> I have determined . . . each year to ascend a few mountains, or at least one . . . for the sake of bodily exercise and the delight of the spirit. For how great the pleasure . . . in wondering at the

mighty mass of mountains while . . . gazing on their immensity
and as it were lifting one's head among the clouds.

A famous early climb was Petrarch's ascent of Mont Ventoux in 1335, a relatively easy climb. More difficult was that of Mont Aiguille by Antoine De Ville, Lord of Domp Julian, in 1492. This spectacular pillar, rising alone a mile high above the plain, was not climbed again, because it is so difficult, for 350 years. Cortez sent his conquistadors to the summit of Popocatépetl (5,366 meters; 17,887 feet) in 1521, not for sport but, it is said, to bring back sulfur for gunpowder.

We do know that there was traffic over alpine passes several centuries ago. Josias Simler, an innkeeper, wrote a mountain guidebook in 1574 detailing routes, recommending clothing, and including sketches of remarkable ice axes and iron claws which travellers should use. Simler described the danger of cold but did not mention mountain sickness.

At the end of the sixteenth century a Jesuit missionary to South America, José de Acosta, wrote his now famous account of the problems he encountered while crossing the high Andean passes. Crossing a high pass called Pariacaca (4,500 meters; 15,000 feet) he wrote:

I was suddenly surprised with so mortall and strange a pang, that I was ready to fall from the top to the ground . . . with such pangs of straining and casting as I thought to cast up my heart too; for having cast up meat, fleugme, and choler . . . if this had continued, I should undoubtedly have died.

Best known are the ascents of Mont Blanc, the highest peak in Europe, in 1789 and the more formidable Matterhorn (4,407 meters; 14,690 feet) a century later. But mountaineering for sport did not become popular until the middle of the nineteenth century, when, in a span of thirty years, all the alpine summits were reached, and thousands of men and a few women, excited by Dr. Albert Smith's illustrated lectures, took up the sport. Climbers everywhere described the symptoms even before lack of oxygen was shown to be the cause; the symptoms were so common that failure to describe them might cast doubt on the climber's achievement. Almost exactly a century later the golden age of Himalayan climbing began, and today most of the world's major summits have been reached. But thousands of others, unmapped, many still unseen, remain to beckon.

3. GOING HIGHER

For much the same reason that prompted Philip of Macedon to climb Mount Haemus, men must have looked to the heavens wondering how far they could see if they went up to a higher place. Was space infinite or did it end abruptly? What might lie beyond? An old Chinese saying held that the tops of two sacred mountains, Wugong and Taibei, "are only 300 feet to the sky." Venus, the evening star, was called the Taibei star because she was thought to live on that summit.

Early Flight

For millennia men have envied birds gliding out of sight and have longed to be free of Earth. As the Aristotelian dogma defining the atmosphere crumbled, scientists discovered the true nature of air and space. Some wondered if it might not be possible to travel in this environment much as Beeckman said, "like a fish in water." Around 1508 Leonardo da Vinci patterned wings after those of birds, which a man might flap and use to fly. Although we do not know if these were actually tested in the sixteenth century, they have been repeatedly tried since, even today.

In the seventeenth century Laurenco de Guzmao patented an extraordinary airship called the *Passarola* of which only his drawing survives. He must have appreciated the lifting power of hot air, because in 1709 he filled a small parchment globe with air from the "combustion of various quintessences" and flew it in the King of Portugal's palace. It rose to the ceiling and set fire to the draperies. Although "his majesty was good enough not to take it ill," there was talk of sorcery, and Guzmao fled to Toledo where he died in 1724, unhonored and forgotten.

Going on Périer's theory that air was thinner and lighter at higher altitudes, a Dominican friar named Joseph Galien had the ingenious idea of filling a giant airship with air from the top of a high mountain. Just how this would be accomplished was not explained, however. Francesco de Lana-Terzi used Guericke's pump to evacuate thin copper spheres that were supposed to lift off from the Earth, but they were too thin and collapsed under the atmospheric pressure.

Nevertheless, these early ideas suggested that a suitable container, filled with a substance lighter than air, might leave the Earth. Henry Cavendish had already isolated such a substance—hydrogen—with which Tiberias Cavallo filled various bladders (1775 to 1782). But he made little progress; the bladders leaked.

The first real flights were made by the Montgolfier brothers, Joseph-Michel and Jacques-Etienne, of France. In November 1782 they filled a small taffeta balloon with hot air and watched it float to the ceiling of their room, just as Guzmao had done. A few weeks later, in secrecy, they repeated this effort successfully with a larger balloon. Finally on June 4, 1783, before a huge crowd, they released a very large balloon that took off and floated out of sight, landing several miles away. A few months later they used huge balloons, carrying first animals, then a man (Pilatre de Rozier). These balloons were filled with hot smoke from smoldering hay, which limited their lift and the distance they could fly. Within a few months, hydrogen lifted other balloons; however the supply of this rare gas was limited and costly.

Unfortunately, Rozier later tried a combination of hot air and hydrogen. The inflammable gas exploded, whether from sparks from the smoldering hay or from static was disputed. This dampened but did not halt these sensational ventures. Balloons became fashionable: Testu Brissey flew astride a horse, an opera singer' sang arias, and the first airmail was carried across the English Channel.

Hydrogen balloons could go much higher. J.-A.-C. Charles and two brothers, A. J. and F. M Robert, made a new balloon and generated hydrogen at the launching place. Late in 1783 Charles and one of the Robert brothers flew in this to 3,000 meters (10,000 feet) using a Torricellian barometer as an altimeter. They noticed no adverse symptoms. Shortly thereafter the intrepid Jean Piérre Blanchard claimed to have reached 9,600 meters (32,000 feet) where he fell into a deep sleep but somehow survived. Joseph Gay-Lussac counted his pulse and respirations at 6,600 meters (22,000 feet) just as De Saussure was doing on Mont Blanc. He claimed to notice no inconvenience at that dangerous altitude.

In 1862 Henry Coxwell and James Glaisher made a number of high altitude flights, narrowly escaping death on one occasion when they may have gone as high as 8,700 meters (29,000 feet). Glaisher made so many high flights that he claimed to have developed a tolerance. With remarkable prescience he wrote, "At length I became acclimatized to the effects of a more rarefied atmosphere." Here is the first observation of acclimatization since Haidar and Acosta, centuries before.

The Discoveries of Bert

With the popularity of ballooning and, in the middle of the nineteenth century, alpine climbing, many theories of the cause of mountain sickness were advanced. Conrad Meyer-Ahrens, a leading Zurich physician covered all bases:

> Mountain sickness is due to (a) decrease in the absolute quantity of oxygen, (b) rapidity of evaporation, (c) intensity of light, (d) expansion of intestinal gases and (e) weakening of the coxo-femoral articulation.

Others thought that diminished atmospheric pressure caused the fluids and gases of the body to expand. An American surgeon blamed the Earth's magnetism. Maladjustment of the spine or of the hip joint, or "spinal anemia" due to decreased pressure on the spine was blamed. For centuries emanations from plants (rhubarb, marigold, heather) or minerals (antimony, lead) had been considered responsible.

Unpleasant symptoms were being reported by mountaineers swarming up peaks all over the world when a remarkable French doctor, Paul Bert, began to study the physiological effects of altitude. In 1877 he proved that lack of oxygen was the major, if not the sole, cause of mountain sickness. Bert's encyclopedic book, *Barometric Pressure,* makes him and his colleague, Denis Jourdannet, the true fathers of aviation medicine and major contributors to what we know today about hypoxia.

Bert was fortunate in his friendship with Jourdannet, a wealthy Paris doctor who had made some interesting studies of the blood of natives living at high altitude in Mexico. Together they were a productive partnership, and Jourdannet supported publication of Bert's book. Jourdannet also designed and commissioned an altitude research laboratory for Bert with two steel cylinders as decompression chambers. In these chambers, Bert took animals and himself to simulated high altitudes, noting symptoms similar to those experienced on mountains. His next step was to breathe oxygen from a large leather bag as the chamber was decompressed. This time there were no symptoms. From several such experiments, Bert concluded that lack of oxygen was the cause of mountain sickness and that breathing oxygen would prevent it.

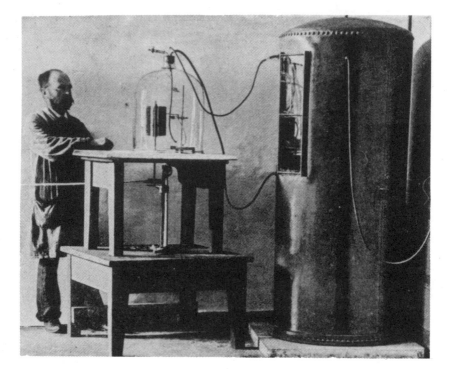

Figure 3-1

Bert's contemporary, an Italian physician named Angelo Mosso, was also studying the effects of altitude, not only in a decompression chamber but in a laboratory atop Monte Rosa, which at 4,561 meters (15,203 feet) is the second highest summit in Europe. Mosso observed the effects of decompression on two young men whose brains could be observed through holes in the skull. He showed that rapid ascent of Monte Rosa could cause an inflammation of the lungs (now recognized as high altitude pulmonary edema). Mosso also observed that at altitude the breathing increased naturally, removing some carbon dioxide from the lungs and blood and thus causing a condition which he named "acapnia." Mosso argued that both lack of oxygen and loss of carbon dioxide caused mountain sickness. Today we recognize that acapnia plays only a small part in mountain sickness.

Two other influences found on high mountains—cold and decreased atmospheric pressure—have been found under some circumstances to contribute to mountain sickness. By the end of the nineteenth century, however, lack of oxygen—then called hypoxemia but now more accurately hypoxia—was established as the major cause.

4. MOVING AIR: VENTILATION

Life as we know it is completely dependent on oxygen. True, there are a few microscopic organisms that live without oxygen, in fact are killed by it, and there may be other forms of life in outer space that might depend on some other element. Most living organisms on Earth, however, require a constant, uninterrupted supply of oxygen most of the time.

Some animals, such as turtles, lungfish, and some insects, are able to adjust their metabolism so they can survive for weeks, months, or even years, anaerobically, that is, without oxygen. This remarkable phenomenon is fascinating and still not completely understood. Other animals, such as bears, ground squirrels, woodchucks, and many others, are able to throttle down their "engines" so they can "sleep," that is, hibernate or aestivate, for months almost without breathing.

Others, notably the diving mammals, can regulate blood flow and oxygen transfer to enable themselves to go for an hour or more without taking in a fresh supply of air. Even you and I spent our first nine months of life in an environment of less than half the oxygen that we need when born.

Once born, however, we, unlike these unusual fellow passengers on Spaceship Earth, require a constant supply of oxygen. If deprived of it for six minutes, our most distinctive feature, the brain, is irreparably damaged. Other functions may continue for minutes or hours. (Hair is said to continue growing for days, even weeks, after death.) After five or six minutes without oxygen, however, we are basically dead. Unlike many other essential substances, we neither store nor make oxygen in our bodies. Nevertheless, as we shall see later, we can, and sometimes do, manage with considerably less than our customary supply, and there are some oxygen stores from which we draw briefly in time of urgent need.

Living organisms have many different breathing apparatuses, but their functions are the same: to supply oxygen to the living cells. All mammals have some sort of pump that takes in fresh air and gets rid of stale air. Oxygen is extracted and waste products, mainly carbon dioxide, are discarded. Fish breathe by passing water through gills where oxygen diffuses into blood; if the water has too little oxygen the fish die. Birds have a rather complicated system of tubes and air sacs and manage to extract more oxygen from air than we can. That is one reason why many birds can fly to heights that would rapidly disable and kill us. Primitive single-celled animals get their oxygen by diffusion.

A hundred years after Christ, Galen systematically described anatomy, physiology, and medical treatment so comprehensively that his doctrine dominated medicine for fifteen hundred years. Galen was trainer and doctor to the gladiators, and he learned his anatomy by treating their wounds and by dissecting animals. Galen drew diagrams of the heart, circulation, and lungs and described how blood and air were moved in the body. Much of what he described was wrong, of course, because the physical properties of the atmosphere were unknown and microscopic anatomy impossible. Though his teaching strangled innovation for many centuries, much of what we know today stems from his insights as well as from his' misconceptions.

Once the weight of air had been demonstrated, and the presence in it of some "vital substance" was established, the next steps came more quickly. John Mayow described breathing very clearly:

> With respect then to the entrance of air into the lungs . . . it is caused by the pressure of the atmosphere. For as the air, on account of the superincumbent atmosphere . . . rushes into all empty places . . . it follows that air passes through the nostrils and the trachea and into the bronchia . . . when the inner sides of the thorax are drawn outwards by muscles . . . and the space in the thorax is enlarged, the air . . . rushes in. From this we conclude that the lungs are distended by the air rushing in and do not expand of themselves, as some have supposed.

He saw that air is not sucked into the lungs but *pushed* in by the atmospheric pressure, an important distinction.

Breathing is the result of the action of small muscles between the ribs, and a large, powerful muscle (the diaphragm). When these muscles contract, the chest expands, increasing the volume of the thorax. As a result outside air is pushed through the nose or mouth where it is warmed and moisturized. It is

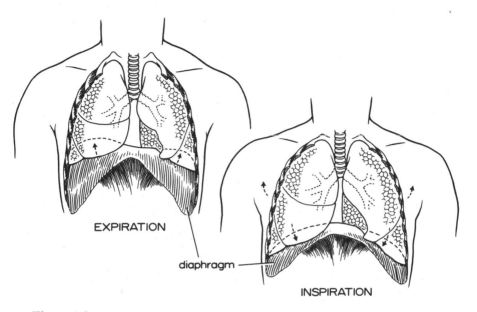

EXPIRATION

diaphragm

INSPIRATION

Figure 4-1

then pushed into the trachea (windpipe) and into smaller and smaller passages (bronchi and bronchioles). Finally, the inrushing air reaches tiny air sacs (alveoli), from which oxygen diffuses into the blood. When we relax the muscles of respiration, the elastic thorax resumes its resting dimensions, and the air in the lungs is forced out by atmospheric pressure on the chest wall, taking with it whatever waste products (mostly carbon dioxide) that have diffused from the blood into the alveoli.

Breathing is actually a very simple, mechanical process. There is nothing magical about it, though our lives depend on its smooth and regularly repeated rhythm. Besides the structure of the respiratory tree, and the mechanics of chest expansion and contraction, the most important part of the process depends on another physical principle—diffusion.

Think of it this way: All walls or barriers have holes between the molecules of which they are made. Lead and iron are quite dense; wood, paper, and cloth much less so. Living membranes are barriers with many holes through which substances may pass. Some membranes have very small holes that allow only small molecules to pass; they are often called semipermeable. (Your raincoat, for example, may allow the small molecules of air to enter and leave but stops the larger molecules of water.)

The membrane walls of the alveoli are semipermeable and so beautifully engineered that oxygen and carbon dioxide and some other small-molecule gases will pass freely, but water, blood, and most substances in blood are halted. The process is called diffusion, and it depends on five factors.

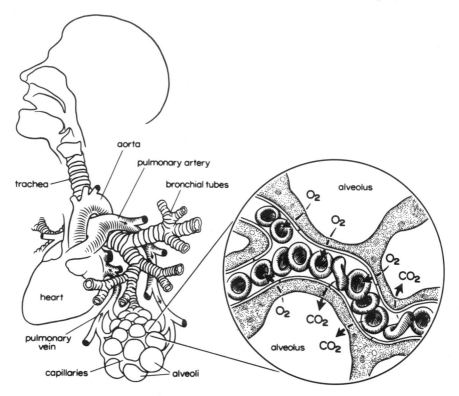

Figure 4-2

First is the nature and area of the membrane. Its permeability and size determine its *diffusion coefficient,* which defines what substances will pass through it and how easily they will do so. Next is the nature of the substance on the other side of the membrane: is it a big molecule (water) or a small one (oxygen)? This defines the diffusion coefficient of the substance. The thickness of the membrane is also important, because the greater the distance a substance must move, the more slowly it diffuses. Then there is the pressure of each substance on either side of the membrane. In the case of a gas this is what Dalton defined as its partial pressure. In the lungs, the partial pressure of oxygen in fresh air is higher than that in the blood on the other side of the alveolar membrane, so oxygen passes through into the blood. For the same reason, carbon dioxide carried to the lungs in the blood has a higher partial pressure in the blood and thus diffuses into the alveoli.

Each of the influences on diffusion is important in respiration (and in virtually all life processes), and each can delay the supply of life-giving oxygen, sometimes seriously. Problems somewhere in the airway from nose and mouth to alveoli are the most important cause of oxygen lack.

At the beginning of the twentieth century a fascinating and heated argument developed between two giants of physiology, John Haldane and Joseph Barcroft. Haldane contended that oxygen could be secreted by the lungs, moving from alveoli into the lung capillaries. This would make the partial pressure of oxygen lower in the alveoli than in the capillaries bringing blood to them. He based his theory on clinical observation and on the fact that after people had stayed at a high altitude for a few days or weeks, the unpleasant symptoms experienced on arrival disappeared.

Though Haldane could not know it, most cells are in fact able to secrete substances, passing them through channels or pores in the cell membrane, uphill as it were, from low pressure inside the cell to higher pressure outside. We will discuss membrane transport when we look more closely at the cell in chapter 7.

Barcroft had no evidence for or against Haldane's theory until he determined to measure simultaneously the partial pressure of oxygen in arterial blood and in alveolar air. Barcroft used a big steel needle, first used by William Stadie, to draw blood from his artery at the moment he exhaled as much air as possible from the depths of his lungs. After several experiments, both in the laboratory and on a high mountain, he showed that the alveolar air always contained more oxygen than did arterial blood coming from the lungs. Haldane clung to his theory for years, however, arguing that acclimatization to altitude depends in part on oxygen secretion. We don't believe this today, but we still need to study people who have become well acclimatized. Perhaps this may show Haldane partly right, although this is unlikely.

We can see that as air enters the body, travels to the alveoli, and then passes into the blood, some of the partial pressure of oxygen is lost at each stage. We call this downhill passage the "oxygen cascade," and the drop continues into the cells. The elimination of carbon dioxide is just as important as the entry of oxygen into the blood, and it moves in obedience to the same laws. The drops in the carbon dioxide cascade are smaller because carbon dioxide diffuses much more readily than does oxygen.

These laws of physics are vitally important. Consider what happens when you double your rate of breathing. More fresh air, rich in oxygen, is pushed into the alveoli, increasing its partial pressure as it mixes with the stale air. Oxygen diffusion into the blood increases. But—an important but—this over-breathing (hyperventilation) also washes more carbon dioxide out of the alveoli, thus decreasing its partial pressure in the blood. Either breathing too much or breathing too little can be extremely significant in health or illness, as we shall see later.

A few other facts must be considered. The air we breathe is often very dry, especially on high mountains. It must not only be warmed but also saturated with water. Otherwise exhaling would drain water from the living cells of the respiratory tree and rapidly dry out the body. After the entering air is fully moisturized, the water vapor, a gas which behaves like every other gas, must be included in the partial pressure equation. Water vapor in fully saturated air at body temperature has a partial pressure of 47 torr at any altitude. The higher we go, the lower the barometric pressure and the lower the partial pressure of oxygen, and the greater the impact of this irreducible 47 torr[1] of water vapor.

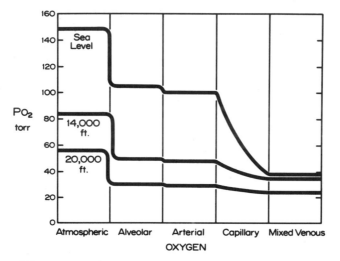

Figure 4-3

Warming the frigid air we breathe on high mountains takes energy, which means it uses oxygen. As incoming air passes through the moist mucus membranes lining our nose, mouth, and windpipe, it is warmed to body temperature and fully saturated with water. In fact, just warming and moisturizing the cold, dry air we breathe on top of Mount Everest (8,796 meters; 29,028 feet) takes so much of our metabolic energy that we cannot stay warm there for more than a short time no matter what we wear. These factors must also be included when we calculate the alveolar oxygen and carbon dioxide pressures.

The alveolar wall that separates the air cell from blood in the lung capillary consists of a layer of tightly joined cells, a tiny space occupied by strands of fibrin called the *interstitial space,* and the double-layered wall of the lung capillary. Gases must diffuse through this thin sandwich. Normally the resistance of this membrane causes only a few torr of pressure decrease, which we call the alveolar-arterial (A-a) gradient. But in many diseases of the

[1]The torr is a unit of measurement equal to the weight of one millimeter of mercury, used to define pressure. It is named for Torricelli.

lung, such as miners' black lung or thickening of the alveolar walls (fibrosis) due to other causes, the A-a oxygen gradient is greatly increased, and the body lacks oxygen as a result. A temporary increase in the gradient affects most of us who go rapidly from low to even moderate altitude because we accumulate a small amount of water in the interstitial space. This increases its resistance and thus the A-a gradient. If this interstitial water is not promptly reabsorbed (as it usually is), it will lead to high altitude pulmonary edema.

We also know that many insults, such as toxic gases, poisons in the blood stream, high blood pressure in the vessels of the lungs, and especially lack of oxygen, change the characteristics of the wall between alveolus and capillary, allowing more fluid, even blood, to pass from one side to the other. It is this change in diffusion characteristics, plus the stretching of the capillary walls, that is a major contributor to edema, as we will see later

Unlike birds and some other animals who move air through the respiratory tract "in one end and out the other," we move air back and forth. This is called the tidal air, and we never get rid of all the residual air deep in the lungs. A battery of tests can describe how well or poorly respiration works. These are collectively known as the Pulmonary Function Tests (PFT), and are shown in figure 1.

They can often define processes that lead to hypoxia or to carbon dioxide accumulation, conditions such as emphysema, asthma, and congestive heart failure, for example.

Breathing is controlled by a sensitive set of feedback loops. Primary control rests in at least two places. One is the respiratory center or centers in the medulla (the midbrain), which respond to changes in the acidity of the blood, which in turn is strongly affected by the level of carbon dioxide. The other control is in two olive-sized organs in the neck, the carotid bodies, which react primarily to changes in the amount of oxygen in blood. An early and important response to lack of oxygen is an increase in ventilation, both in rate and depth, which, as we have seen, brings more outside air deep into the lungs, raising alveolar oxygen pressure and lowering that of carbon dioxide. When carbon dioxide decreases, the blood becomes more alkaline, and this signals the respiratory center in the medulla to decrease ventilation, which has been stimulated by oxygen lack.

For the centers that control breathing, this paradox poses the difficult task of trying to maintain the constancy of the internal environment (homeostasis) in spite of two opposing demands: On the one hand oxygen lack must be relieved by hyperventilation. On the other hand, the acidity (pH) of blood and tissues must be held near normal (7.4), and this is negated by that hyperventilation. Faced with this dilemma, the body compromises by increasing respiration enough to elevate alveolar oxygen, while at the same time excreting bicarbonate in the urine to offset the ventilatory alkalosis. Later we will see how success in balancing these two conflicting demands determines whether or not one is stricken with altitude sickness or acclimatizes successfully.

This dual control of breathing causes an interesting phenomenon, a kind of schizophrenic fluctuation called periodic or Cheyne-Stokes respiration, which is common above 2,400 meters (8,000 feet). (It is also common in the elderly and in many illnesses, especially those in terminal states.) Typically, a period of rapid and increasingly deep breaths is followed by shallower breaths until breathing stops completely for an alarming time, before the cycle repeats. Periodic breathing is more pronounced during sleep, which means that average arterial oxygenation is lower than when awake. Snoring in Cheyne-Stokes rhythm is very alarming.

Breathing is only the first step in the transfer of oxygen from air to the cells that are the real seat of life. Other processes are just as important, but none is free-standing, they depend on each other. The whole process of oxygen transport is affected by the innumerable transfers of fluids, salts, acids, and a myriad of other substances across different membranes. In truth, without diffusion life would be impossible.

5. MOVING BLOOD: CIRCULATION

Breathing in and out would not be very useful without some means by which to carry oxygen from lungs to the cells and to remove carbon dioxide. Wondrous though the process of breathing may be, the circulatory system is even more remarkable.

Central to circulation of course is the heart, celebrated by poets and lovers, but as physiologists know, nothing but a tireless mechanical pump. If it has emotional or spiritual qualities, these have yet to be found, though recently we have learned that the heart does produce at least one substance that stimulates other organs.

Let us first consider the heart as a pump. In an average person leading a placid, undisturbed, and inactive life for seventy-five years, the heart will beat some 276 million times and pump about 47 million gallons of blood. In our real lives, with their periods of excitement, exertion, and stress, these figures are likely to be more than half again higher.

What is even more spectacular is the fact that the heart can, if necessary, beat at its own intrinsic rate, unaffected by any stimuli from elsewhere in the body, as long as it receives an adequate inflow of blood carrying oxygen and nutrients, and as long as wastes like carbon dioxide are carried away. Knowing this, we should not be surprised that the properly sheltered heart, removed from the body, may be able to beat almost indefinitely; indeed hearts from some animals have done so. This independence is made possible by a small natural pacemaker called the sino-atrial node, located in the wall of the right atrium (one of the four chambers of the heart).

From this phenomenal little electric generator, nerves lead to the heart muscle carrying the tiny impulse that makes the muscle contract or allows it to relax. This independence is rarely needed, but it does make possible successful heart transplants since all nerves to and from the heart are severed by the operation.

Its very independence also makes the heart indispensable. Humans can live for weeks, or months, even for years, with little brain activity, and for days or weeks with deficient kidney, digestive, and hormonal functions. But let the heart stop pumping blood for a mere five or six minutes and first the brain and then other organs are irreversibly damaged and quickly die. An active and effective heart, or a mechanical substitute, must pump blood day in and day out without interruption for us to survive.

From the higher centers in the brain come nervous impulses caused by excitement, anger, pain, or fear—what we might call the love, fight, or flee responses. Receptors in the skin sensitive to temperature may signal the brain to send orders to increase or decrease the heart rate; other centers may give instructions to glands of internal secretion, the adrenals, for example, to release the powerful stimulant adrenaline and its analogs. Veteran race horses greatly increase both rate and output of the heart in anticipation, many seconds before the start of a race. We also do this as we anticipate a difficult or dangerous interview or task, well before the need actually arises.

Under most circumstances throughout our lives the heart is driven by one or several of four major stimuli: nervous, hormonal, blood volume, and the internal environment of the body (temperature, acidity, and chemistry).

Both the parasympathetic and sympathetic nervous systems affect the heart. The receptors in the carotid bodies in the neck stimulate not only breathing; they also affect how much blood the heart pumps. On arrival at altitude, the heart beats faster and more forcefully, putting out more blood per stroke and per minute. This increased cardiac output continues for a few days during the stay at altitude before falling to, or slightly below normal, replaced by the other adjustments (acclimatization) which we will consider in chapter 9. Blood pressure is likely to increase in many people after a few days at altitude.

The heart pumps out what it receives: if blood volume is decreased by hemorrhage or dehydration, for example, the cardiac output will decrease. But if too much blood enters the heart, output will also fall, in compliance with the "law of the heart" developed by British physiologist Ernest Starling almost a century ago. This "law of diminishing returns" applies to many other processes too.

There are other subtle influences on the heart. Strenuous exertion increases the heart rate even before the biochemical changes from working muscles are felt. Impulses from the stomach and intestines, working through changes in the blood, affect the heart. After a heavy meal the rate and output may increase, but after a light meal the rate may slow; in either situation sleep becomes tempting.

We are mainly interested in the effects of altitude. The carotid bodies will stimulate the heart to beat faster and a bit harder above 1,500 meters (5,000 feet). The work of climbing further increases the rate and strength of the heartbeat, and at higher elevations may push the heart beyond its capacity to respond. This may limit work by older people, whose maximal achievable heart rate can be crudely defined as 200 minus half one's age. Maximal breathing capacity also decreases with age, though not predictably. Both of these are discouraging features of aging, but they can be slightly delayed by regular exercise and sensible life-style

Do the heart and the lungs affect the tolerance of the elderly for altitude? We don't have a clear answer to this question, which looms over all of us as the years rush by. Fortunately, ambition is also cooled a bit by age, and many can continue to the end with what they long to do.

We know a great deal about the heart and the blood vessels, which carry blood from the heart to the tissues and back to the heart. Like so much of what we know, however, understanding came by slow steps, sometimes in the wrong direction, until, almost suddenly, someone took a giant stride and reached a new level of understanding from which progress began anew.

Five centuries before Christ a remarkable philosopher-scientist, Empedocles (about whom much myth and some truth have survived) compared the flow of blood to the ebb and flow of the tides. Aristotle took the next step, observing that there were two types of blood, a "spiritual," which was purified by passing through the lungs, and a "venous," which moved through the rest of the body. He was the first to describe the branching of both arteries and veins from large to smaller and smaller, but, like his contemporary, he thought the veins carried blood, while the arteries were filled with *pneuma* or air. He was almost correct. Had he made the simple observations that Fabricius and Harvey made a thousand years later, he might have described how blood actually flows from heart to lungs, from lungs to body, and back to the heart and again to the lungs. But he did not. Instead Aristotle and later Galen taught that there were two separate circulations, and that blood oozed through tiny pores between the two halves of the heart. Galen probably had opportunities to examine human hearts because of his work as doctor to the gladiators, but the microscope which would have helped him was many centuries in the future.

Leonardo da Vinci also recognized that the heart was a pump, but he did not describe the circulation. One who did was Michael Servetus, who in 1550 challenged Galen's dictum, defied the church, was charged with heresy, and burned at the stake. Three copies of his great book survived the purge and show that he had correctly figured out the path of the blood, though he had no way to demonstrate this experimentally.

In 1924 manuscripts written by a fourteenth-century Persian physician, Ibn-al-Nafis, were discovered. He stated that the blood followed the course we know today, and that the purpose of the lungs was to purify the blood. His theory was remarkable, not only because his religious faith prevented dissection, but also because the discovery of oxygen was still five centuries in the future. In 1524 another pioneer, Renaldo Colummbo, was teaching the correct pathways of blood. Undoubtedly others now long forgotten, among them Andreas Cesalpino, were also on the right path.

William Harvey deserves honor, not because he made a great new discovery, but because he had the genius to put together the observations of others, eloquently but simply describing how the circulation of humans and most animals works. He buttressed his argument by calculating that in one hour the heart pumped blood weighing more than three times the weight of the entire body. His synthesis was so masterful that it seemed no one could challenge him, but old beliefs die hard, and he was harshly attacked at home and abroad. Though stung, he refused to respond. Most of his contemporaries supported him, and he won acceptance from those who mattered most. Harvey was physician to James I and later to Charles I. In 1628, prefaced with a letter to King Charles, he published his famous book *De Motu Cordis,* in which he wrote:

> Since calculations and visual observations have confirmed all my suspicions, to wit that the blood is passed through the lungs and the heart by the pulsations of the ventricles, is forcibly ejected to all parts of the body, therein steals into the veins and the porosities of the flesh, flows everywhere back through those very veins from the circumference to the center, from small veins into larger ones, and thence comes at last into the vena cava and to the auricle of the heart . . . I am forced to conclude that . . . the blood is driven around with an unceasing circular sort of movement.

Four years after his death, Malpighi of Pisa, using the newly developed microscope, was able to see the tiny capillaries (which Harvey called "porosities") and to confirm Harvey's speculations. With this demonstration Harvey's description of the continuity of the vessels that carry blood throughout the body was confirmed.

Experiments with the heart and blood vessels multiplied. Stephen Hales, a clergyman better known for his pioneer studies of plant respiration, inserted a thin tube into the carotid artery of a horse and measured blood pressure for the first time; he may have done so in a man as well. He described the capacity of the heart as a pump, and from this and the pulse rate accurately calculated how much blood was pumped per minute—the first definition of the cardiac output. A hundred and fifty years later two French physiologists, Auguste Chauveau and Jules Marey, took another giant stride: devising a double-chambered tube (catheter) which they passed through a vein into the right side of the heart, they measured the cardiac output of horses.

Until the twentieth century measurements on arterial blood were limited to animals, or obtained by slashing an artery; neither method was satisfactory for studies of the dynamics of respiration and circulation. During an epidemic of pneumonia in 1916, William Stadie wished to see whether the amount of oxygen in blood might predict the outcome in serious cases. Through a small cut in the skin he inserted a needle into an artery, drew blood, and measured the oxygen content. Ten years later, Joseph Barcroft used this same type of needle to draw arterial blood at the same time he obtained alveolar air. He measured the oxygen in the two samples and showed that the lungs were not capable of secreting oxygen into the blood, pushing it uphill as Haldane claimed. Arterial punctures are commonplace today, but the needles are much more refined.

I had a brief encounter with another advance which did me no credit. I was finishing my residency training in Presbyterian Hospital in New York when two men asked if they might do an experiment on one of my patients. Appalled by what they told me, I indignantly refused, saying I couldn't see any use whatever in what they wanted to do, and they went elsewhere. Both of them—Andre Cournand and Dickinson Richards, later became my close friends and teachers.

What Cournand and Richards proposed was to repeat an experiment first tried in 1929 when a young German surgeon, Werner Forssmann, pushed a thin, flexible catheter (much like the one Hales had used on a horse two hundred years before), through his veins into his own heart, watching the process displayed on a fluoroscope. Cournand and Richards perfected the instrument and technique and were able to measure not only the dynamics within the heart but the flow and pressure within the pulmonary artery and the small vessels of the lung as well. Through this technique doctors gained an intimate understanding of the effects of hypoxia on the circulation of the lung, a factor that is immensely important in understanding altitude sickness.

6. THE VITAL FLUID

What means would you use to carry oxygen from lungs to the cells throughout the body? In what sort of vehicle? Would you dissolve oxygen in the blood? Oxygen is very soluble in many liquids. Would a chemical combination be better? Oxygen combines either strongly or weakly with most substances. Should the transporter be alive or an inert, unchanging material, and how should it be contained? Each of these questions has been explored but no means has yet been found to improve on the system we were born with and which works for so many animals.

We, like most mammals, use small single cells to carry oxygen. Smaller than a grain of sand, the human red blood cell is shaped roughly like a rubbery pancake, slightly flattened in the middle. Enclosed in a thin, permeable membrane is a watery substance packed with a complex molecule, and a few enzymes. Oxygen combines with hemoglobin loosely, so that it is responsive to slight changes in the partial pressure of oxygen in its surrounding liquid. On the average men and women have 4.5 to 5.0 million red blood cells in each milliliter of blood, a total of about 25 billion in an adult.

Most animals, fish, birds, mammals, and many others, use a complex protein containing iron to combine reversibly with oxygen. It is a four-part molecule, formed by the interlocking of two pairs of different kinds of hemoglobin. Usually this quartet is contained within the red blood cell, but in some species it is in simple solution.

Red cells live—perhaps survive is a better word—for three or four months, but during that time they are in constant motion, carried to every nook and cranny, unloading oxygen in the capillaries, returning to the heart and thence to the lungs where they are reloaded with oxygen only to continue their unceasing round. Not surprisingly they wear out, and are destroyed or recycled, mostly in the spleen, which also serves as a garage for holding some reserve blood for time of crisis. New red blood cells are constantly being made in the bone marrow, to be released as needed. Their formation is stimulated by a hormone called erythropoietin (red making), which orders the marrow to make hemoglobin and to insert it into some primitive stem cells that seem to hang around waiting to serve.

Fortunately for mountaineers, lack of oxygen at high altitude, as in certain illnesses, is a very powerful stimulus, causing erythropoietin to increase almost instantly so red cell production is driven to respond to the need. Red cell formation is delicately adjusted: the more severe the oxygen lack, the more hemoglobin and red cells are made. But only to a certain amount: red cell production usually levels off about 40 to 50 percent above normal no matter how high one goes or how severe the hypoxia.

The red cells are carried in a kind of broth, the plasma, which is rich in all sorts of substances. Plasma contains many proteins, fats, and different types of carbohydrate, not in their original form, but digested to their component amino acids, fatty acids, and simple sugars. Hormones and enzymes are also transported in plasma, along with calcium, potassium, and sodium in different combinations, and many trace elements. An extraordinary set of materials regulate blood clotting, and when blood is clotted it leaves a clear yellowish liquid called serum.

Only a little oxygen is dissolved in blood; most is carried in combination with hemoglobin. On the other hand, carbon dioxide dissolves readily, and most of it is carried from tissues to lungs in solution or combined in buffer pairs that control the acidity of blood. Many hormones, enzymes, and other substances carried in blood are involved in maintaining the constancy of our internal environment, defending us from infection, acquiring nutrients, and rejecting wastes. We will consider only the principal function of the red cells, which is the carriage of oxygen to, and carbon dioxide from, cells to lungs.

Our knowledge of blood is extensive, but new interactions and new substances are continually being found. Some substances occur in extremely tiny amounts but are persistent and powerful; others form in response to certain influences and rapidly vanish. Many materials move through capillary walls, but many others do not, except under special conditions. The passage of molecules through capillary walls and through the cell membranes is a major, complex, and fascinating subject. Although primarily a transport vehicle, blood and its contents affect every living function.

As always we find that the ancients had some understanding and great respect for blood. Our friend Empedocles wrote, "The blood is life," and Aristotle considered blood the soul of man. Galen corrected his predecessors by showing that arteries carried "pure" blood, while veins carried "impure" blood, which is not so far from the truth!

It would be two thousand years before the circulatory system was understood much more clearly, and it took even longer to recognize all the other functions of blood. Only after the microscope was made could Anthony van Leeuwenhoeck (one of those with a strong claim to having made the first one) write in 1674: "I have observed, taking some blood from my hand, that it consists of small round globules driven through a crystalline humidity of water."

A few years before Leeuwenhoeck gave his address to the Royal Society, Richard Lower noticed that when blood was shaken with air it turned a brighter scarlet than when allowed to stand. John Hooke found that dogs could be kept alive, even if their chests were opened, as long as air was pumped in and out of the lungs. In another hundred years the explanation was made clear by the isolation of oxygen and the demonstration of how essential it was to life.

The Oxyhemoglobin Dissociation Curve

In yet another century Paul Bert designed the instrument that enabled him to define the relationship between hemoglobin and the partial pressure of oxygen, what we know today as the oxyhemoglobin dissociation curve. This curve describes what percentage of hemoglobin will carry oxygen when blood is exposed to different partial pressures of oxygen, and its shape is crucial to the acquisition and release of oxygen by blood.

The normal dissociation curve in humans is S-shaped. This means it will pick up oxygen easily and will be almost completely loaded (96 to 98 percent saturated) over a wide range of oxygen pressure in the lungs. It also means that hemoglobin holds onto oxygen strongly until, in the tissues, the oxygen pressure falls quite low, whereupon oxygen is released with a rush. Venous blood, flowing back to the lungs for reloading, will have a partial pressure of oxygen at or below 40 torr and be less than 70 percent saturated.

Fascinating though this is in the laboratory, in the living animal it is little short of miraculous. The S shape is ideal for its function, and it is affected by events in such a way as to maxi"mize its effectiveness. In life we do not see one nice smooth dissociation curve, but one that is shifted—to the left in the lungs where carbon dioxide is released and to the right in the tissue capillaries where carbon dioxide enters. These shifts make possible more rapid loading and unloading of oxygen. The curve is also distorted at higher altitudes by the loss of carbon dioxide caused by the increased breathing and by the loss of bicarbonate in urine, thus making the blood more alkaline and shifting the curve toward the left. Strenuous exertion releases more carbon dioxide to tissues, as well as some metabolic acids, thus flattening the curve (shifting it to the right) and releasing more oxygen. Despite a vast amount of study, oxygen transport and release still hides some secrets, and some concepts are disputed. What is clear is that the carriage of oxygen by hemoglobin is wonderfully complex.

From the preceding brief description it is clear that we cannot neglect carbon dioxide because it is such an essential ingredient of blood for two big reasons. First, it must be continuously removed as a waste product of cell activity and discarded through the lungs, and without this disposal life would rapidly deteriorate and end. Second, carbon dioxide combines chemically with water and with some proteins in blood to form buffers that soften the impact of changes in the alkalinity or acidity of blood. In our enthusiasm for oxygen it is easy to forget that reliable transport of carbon dioxide is just as crucial to our life and well-being as that of oxygen.

Exploration of the acid-base equilibrium was not productive until the development of instruments to monitor precisely the hydrogen ion concentration of blood and tissues, and most of this delicate work has been done in the last fifty years!

Types of Hemoglobin

There are hundreds of different forms of human hemoglobin and even more in the rest of the animal world. The one of greatest importance to us, one that is indispensable to life, is called *fetal hemoglobin.* From its early life, the fetus synthesizes this primitive type of hemoglobin because it lives and develops in an oxygen atmosphere much like that on the highest Himalayan summits. The partial pressure of oxygen in the mother's placenta, from which oxygen diffuses into the fetal circulation, averages only 50 torr and falls steeply in crossing the membranes between the placenta and the fetal blood.

To protect against such severe oxygen lack, the hemoglobin of the fetus is shifted toward the left so that it grabs oxygen more avidly and releases it less readily, but more rapidly when it does. The fetus has more hemoglobin for its body weight than it will after birth, and there is less carbon dioxide in fetal blood—both factors which improve the carriage of oxygen. Soon after birth F-hemoglobin changes to a transitional form and within a year to the normal adult form, A-hemoglobin.

These wonders are not only of academic interest: without this exuberant transport mechanism the human fetus might not survive. It is not surprising to learn that the changes we see in acclimatization to higher altitudes are similar to those in the fetus: a leftward shift of teh oxygen-hemoglobin dissociation curve, an increased amount of hemoglobin, and decreased amount of carbon dioxide. But adults do not develop a fetal form of hemoglobin on high mountains.

Some altitude-resident animals have done so, however. The barheaded goose, often seen flying at 9,000 meters (30,000 feet) between India and Tibet, and the Andean goose, its distant cousin, do have a hemoglobin genetically different from that of their lowland relatives. So does the deer mouse who lives high in the Sierra, compared to his cousin in Death Valley. The exact sites of change in the amino acid sequence in hemoglobin have been located, making it theoretically possible to create these changes deliberately.

Some individuals are born with hemoglobins whose dissociation curves are left-shifted, much like that of the fetus and the barheaded goose. These mutant forms come in different shapes, and some are incompatible with life. One might predict that people with a mutant hemoglobin that had a higher affinity for oxygen, that is, which was left-shifted, might adjust better to altitude. One study of two adolescents with a left-shifted form of hemoglobin showed that they did in fact adjust to moderate altitude better than did their two siblings who had normal adult hemoglobin.

Mutant hemoglobins may be more important to the millions of people with some defect in lungs or blood that causes severe hypoxia even at sea level. Genetic engineering is evolving very rapidly and may enable us to change the hemoglobin in the fetus when a dangerous mutant has been detected early. Already a chemical has been found that can change one abnormal form, S-hemoglobin, to the normal form, even after birth, but the present formulation seems to cause cancer.

Actually we already have in our bodies what might be called a mutant, the form of hemoglobin that resides only in muscle—myoglobin. Its dissociation curve is sharply left-shifted, so that myoglobin picks up oxygen from the muscle's blood supply, holds it tenaciously, and then, when the partial pressure in tissue falls very low, releases a lot of oxygen rapidly. What better method for meeting the urgent needs of sudden or strenuous muscular effort! Myoglobin is only slightly affected by changes in the carbon dioxide content or acidity of the blood. We might think of myoglobin as a temporary storehouse for oxygen, which can be drawn on during hard physical work.

One of the mutant hemoglobins, the S-, or sickle-form, can cause real problems. Sickle cells are more short-lived than normal blood cells. Because of this, about 0.3 percent of Americans with this form have sickle-cell anemia; another 8-10 percent have the sickle-cell trait. S-hemoglobin has a slightly different molecular configuration than the normal form. S-hemoglobin deforms some of the usually flabby red blood cells into sharp-ended, rigid shapes that have a nasty tendency to stick in capillary walls. The deformity is made worse by lack of oxygen. Not surprisingly, some people with sickle-cell trait may not do well at even moderate altitudes and may develop obstructions in the small vessels of the spleen, muscles, and other organs causing what are called sickle-cell crises.

The sickle-cell trait occurs only in people with African or Mediterranean ancestry, but even a remote ancestor can affect someone today, as this recent report shows:

> An eighteen-year-old man flew from sea level to 7,000 feet and in a few hours was hospitalized because of abdominal pain. Three days later the pain had localized in the area of his spleen. This was removed, sickle-cell damage was found, and he was given oxygen with complete recovery. His father rushed to the hospital during the surgery, developed a similar pain, and his spleen, too, was removed and found damaged by sickle cells. Both were white, but the father later acknowledged the possibility of distant black or Mediterranean ancestry.

Oxygen in the Blood

Under the right conditions, when breathing air at sea level pressure, from 97 to 98 percent of our hemoglobin molecules are loaded with oxygen. This is the oxygen *capacity* of blood, that is, the amount of oxygen, usually measured in volumes of oxygen contained in 100 milliliters of blood (volumes percent). When at high altitude, or when breathing less than the 21 percent of oxygen in air, blood is less fully saturated, and on a high mountain may have only three fourths of what it can carry. We call this the oxygen *content,* also measured in volumes percent. The distinction between capacity and content is important because content can be changed by changing either atmospheric pressure or percentage of oxygen inhaled, but capacity depends on the amount and type of hemoglobin present.

As it is pumped from the heart into the large arteries, onwards to smaller ones, and finally to thin-walled capillaries (which are barely large enough to admit the disc-shaped red cells one at a time), blood loses almost no oxygen. Why? Because blood cells have little metabolic activity. The only other function of red blood cells is to convert carbon dioxide to bicarbonate buffers, influenced by an important enzyme, carbonic anhydrase, which we will discuss later. Hemoglobin pairs also buffer against changes in the acidity of blood. Thus, oxygen content is not changed since oxygen does not leak through the larger vessel walls.

In the capillaries, however, oxygen flows from the high partial pressure in blood to the low pressure in the loose tissues around cells and thence through the cell wall to supply the cell. This passage is controlled by the laws of diffusion described earlier. As oxygen goes in one direction, carbon dioxide (plentiful in cells and tissue, lower in blood) moves in the opposite direction, and in doing so, pushes a bit more oxygen out, a very convenient effect.

Without pause, the red cells continue through the capillaries, into the tiniest veins and so on back to the heart where blood is pumped to the lungs, through thick-walled arteries, and to capillaries. There, where oxygen is high in the alveolus and the venous oxygen is low, red cells pick up oxygen, release carbon dioxide, and continue back to the heart. What is so wonderful is that diffusion is rapid enough in both lungs and tissues that these transfers are scarcely if at all impaired even when the heart is pumping very fast, or very slowly.

The mountaineer may ask another question. High on a great mountain would it help to have more blood, more red cells—say by receiving a transfusion? This would certainly increase the oxygen *capacity* and therefore the oxygen *content*. The few experiments which have been done suggest that the benefit is small, first because the body is constantly making more red cells, second because transfused red cells do not carry a full load of oxygen, having lost some of this capability in storage, and third because transfusions, even of the individual's own blood, can initiate other responses than those we want. Also, since dehydration thickens blood in the high, dry air, adding more red cells in addition to what the body is producing may make the blood too thick to circulate effectively, increasing the risk of blood clotting.

Would the patient with an illness causing hypoxia at sea level benefit from transfusions? Here the answer depends entirely on the cause: the patient who is anemic will certainly benefit by the addition of more red cells. One whose blood lacks oxygen because the lungs are sick and don't allow normal diffusion, will benefit little, and if the hypoxia is due to a failing heart, added blood is more likely to harm than help.

The manufacture of hemoglobin depends on an adequate supply of iron in the body. Most of us get plenty in our diets, but if there is a deficiency, then, but only then, will taking extra iron or certain vitamins make a difference. It may make you feel good to pop iron and vitamins on a high mountain, but there is not much scientific evidence that it helps, although women do sometimes lack iron and need the supplements. Habitual strenuous exercise causes anemia in some men and women, but this exercise anemia does not benefit much from added iron. You must be a real fanatic to develop exercise anemia.

Other Components of Blood

Blood is far more than a carrier of red cells and oxygen. Several other cells have functions that are just as essential to health and life. Blood carries a variety of white blood cells, some of which are scavengers, while others (lymphocytes) fight disease. One family of lymphocytes includes specialized cells that make antibodies against infections and against almost every foreign substance that enters the blood. Helper T-cells and killer T-cells are part of this process, which has become familiar to us because of their role in HIV infection and AIDS. The whole group of autoimmune disturbances is a vast area to explore. There are suggestions that tolerance or intolerance for altitude, and some of the family of altitude illnesses, may be affected by changes in the autoimmune system, an exciting field for study.

Platelets, another of the formed elements in blood, have a vital role in blood clotting. Think of this for a moment: To survive we must have a liquid that is thin enough to move swiftly, yet which must carry literally hundreds of substances that affect its fluidity. This liquid must remain liquid in the body, yet must instantly clot or coagulate when a leak occurs from a broken blood vessel either within or to the outside of the body. We must have a mechanism that prevents clotting when we don't need it, but facilitates clotting when we do. It is a near miracle that only a few relatively rare diseases affect this intricate system. Altitude does alter the clotting mechanism: sometimes platelets are decreased at altitude, and blood clots less readily. But, as we shall see later, in high altitude pulmonary edema the activity of platelets, and the coagulation of blood in the lungs, may be increased or decreased in different individuals.

Blood also transports hormones, messengers made in special glands which speed to their targets to incite appropriate response. Adrenaline and its relatives are well known: fear, anger, and other major stresses cause the adrenal glands (which nestle around each kidney) to shoot this powerful substance into the bloodstream to strengthen the fight or flee response. Dozens of other glands are constantly working, or ready to work, to maintain the stability of our internal environment. Some regulate growth, others control metabolism, the formation of urine, the development of the ovum in women and sperm in men, the appropriate release of enzymes or ferments into the right parts of our digestive system, and many more processes. Special substances formed in the brain cause pleasure and relief of pain; they are called endorphins because they are so similar to morphine and other opium derivatives. More of these special messengers, which occur in very tiny amounts, are being identified every day. Some exist for only a very short time before doing their duties and being converted or destroyed.

This wonderful field of study is dazzling in its size and potential. Already there is considerable evidence that many hormones and enzymes (the two are hard to differentiate, and need better names) are actively involved in our response to altitude and other causes of oxygen lack. For several decades we have been able, by affecting the enzyme carbonic anhydrase, to decrease the symptoms of mountain sickness. One thing is certain: these biologically active substances, even in microscopic amounts, affect everything we do and are important to mountaineers.

Blood also protects us by maintaining our body temperature within a very narrow range regardless of the outside environment. By being shifted to one area or another, blood flow will warm those areas that are chilled or cool those that are overheated. Blood is a vehicle for water, carrying it from the stomach and intestines throughout the body, dumping excess into the sweat or urine, and evaporating some in the nose, mouth, and airways to humidify the air we breathe.

The physiologist Claude Bernard taught Paul Bert and to some extent is responsible for his interest in high altitude. We are continually reminded of Bernard's statement: "The constancy of the internal environment is the condition of a free life." Blood is the key means of maintaining this constancy and makes possible all of our activities. It is the stuff of miracles.

7. CELLS: THE ULTIMATE USERS

Moving air and moving blood have only two purposes, if we may speak teleologically: to sustain and protect living cells. We breathe to provide oxygen and to remove carbon dioxide. The heart pumps hemoglobin-laden blood to carry nourishment to the cells and to remove wastes. Both functions also protect the body's temperature and humidity. If either respiration or circulation fails for more than a few minutes, life ends and cells break up.

Cells are the blocks from which an organism is built, but unlike bricks they are growing, changing, busily functioning units that live and die and replace themselves. There are thousands of varieties of cells with different skills, every one of them originating from the union of two single cells, the sperm and the egg, which carry the genetic messages that define every aspect of the individual. As adults we are made of 75 to 100 trillion cells of many different kinds and functions.

Cells are held together in various structures that define the various parts of the body (spleen, liver, heart, and bone, for example). Each part is built of its unique type of cells, but all are bathed in a common liquid, the extracellular fluid by which their surroundings are kept stable within very narrow limits. We are made of much more water than of solid stuffs, and the constancy of our cells' environment is assured by the extracellular fluid.

Membrane Transport

Though cells with different specialties are somewhat different internally, all (except red blood cells) consist of a rich soup contained in a thin skin. The soup is watery, and contains hundreds of items. These include ions such as sodium, potassium, calcium, and small amounts of others, all of which may pass through channels or pores in the delicate membrane which walls the cell. Many of these ions are constantly being pumped between the intracellular and the extracellular fluid by a bioelectric process called membrane transport. This is an invisible high-energy pump which can actively move selected ions from an area of low concentration to one where it is higher. Certain molecules, such as oxygen and carbon dioxide, pass in and out of cells by simple diffusion. This type of transport is called passive, and is controlled by the laws of diffusion. Breakdown compounds from the food we eat, and other substances secreted or formed by the body, pass the membrane by more elaborate processes called assisted, or active, transport.

Active membrane transport is energy intensive and requires a good bit of oxygen. This is where the cell is particularly vulnerable and one reason why some of us hypothesize that hypoxia impairs the pump and thus alters cell functions.

Because it determines what stays in and what stays out, the structure of the cell wall is as important as its contents. It is a very thin, elastic membrane with six micro-layers, each one molecule thick. From the outside inward it is made of mucopolysaccharides or sugarlike compounds, then several kinds of protein, then fatty substances (lipids), and then a reverse of the outer layer of molecules. Active membrane transport occurs only through specific channels, and how these molecules line up determines where these channels are. Other molecules in the cell wall are responsible only for assisted membrane transport, handing certain substances across the wall as it were. The structure of this membrane, and its functions, are extremely important to life and powerfully affect how well or poorly we tolerate an alien environment such as high altitude.

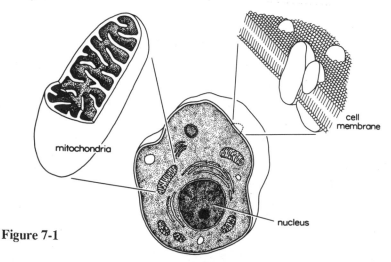

Figure 7-1

The Krebs Cycle

The cell's work is done in many tiny "factories" called mitochondria. Each contains many enzymes which recognize and act upon specific fuel particles that have entered the cell. Each is deeply furrowed or convoluted, and we can picture each as a set of shelves in a chemical laboratory, each shelf crowded with enzymes ready to work. Enzymes are not consumed by the work—they are merely facilitators—"burning" food stuffs to produce carbon dioxide, water, and other products, and releasing energy. How is this possible?

Two centuries ago the discovery of oxygen was followed by demonstrations that most materials would burn when air containing oxygen was available. Burning released heat and light, sometimes a great deal of heat very rapidly. Gradually it was recognized that food was burned by the body much as a candle burns—providing there is a good supply of oxygen. The nagging question then became: how can this happen without torching the body?

In the first half of the nineteenth century, Justus Liebig developed equations to support the concept that sugars are "burned" gradually and slowly in the tissues, not in the blood, to produce carbon dioxide and water. Louis Pasteur built on this by suggesting some similarity between his fermentation studies and the "burning" of sugars in the body. At the end of the nineteenth century Hans and Edward Buchner isolated the substance in yeast that causes fermentation; from this phenomenon (which had been known since Noah!) came the word *enzyme,* meaning "in yeast."

Liebig's concept was refined and tested, and finally in the 1920s Hans Krebs described the elaborate biochemical process called the Krebs (or citric acid) cycle in his honor. This cycle is a series of biochemical reactions, each moving from raw material toward end product, each releasing heat and energy. The heat is carried away by the blood, keeping us warm without burning us up. The released energy does the work, whether it is contracting a muscle fiber, making and releasing a hormone, or initiating digestion. The speed of these processes is controlled by different enzymes and by the availability of fuel. When we starve, the tissues begin to consume themselves; as the fuel supply dwindles, heat and energy decrease, and finally we die.

Something similar happens when we are deprived of adequate oxygen: heat and energy generation decrease, and over time, if oxygen is not provided, we collapse, grow cold, and die, even though food may be there waiting to be used. This is the danger in extreme high altitude climbing.

Responses to Lack of Oxygen

The citric acid cycle requires oxygen and runs as long as fuel and oxygen are available. Two sources for sudden, brief bursts of energy are available. They are called anaerobic because they do not demand oxygen immediately, but they may run up an oxygen debt which must be soon repaid. One, the phosphagen cycle, can instantly produce a large amount of energy for a few seconds, perhaps enough to run a hundred-yard dash, but the cycle, like the runner, is then exhausted. The second, which is based on muscle glycogen (a kind of sugar), can also be activated rapidly. It produces two or three times as much energy as the Krebs cycle, but lasts only one or two minutes. Anaerobic work using either cycle is possible for only a very short time, and so far no way has been found that will allow us to work without oxygen for very long. However, the process of acclimatization does help the cell to get along on a smaller oxygen budget.

Intensive searches have been made for a respiratory enzyme, one that could facilitate the use of oxygen within the cells. Many have been tried, among them the cytochrome family, but this field is far too complex and changing too rapidly for discussion here. We can say with confidence that many enzymes within the cell activate metabolism. Possibly, just possibly, one may be found that will improve tolerance for hypoxia, and which might be given for that purpose to patients chronically hypoxic from disease.

How else do cells acclimatize or adjust to lack of oxygen? Possibly by forming more mitochondria in essential cells, though this has not been proven. We have learned that mitochondria enlarge after prolonged residence at altitude. There is a suggestion too that they move closer to the cell wall, perhaps to be closer to the incoming oxygen.

In fact, however, such changes may be unnecessary and even ineffective. Why? Because the oxygen tension within the cells appears to be very low, probably near 1 or 2 torr. The cell is more likely to acclimatize to altitude by using more enzymes for more efficient, or even new pathways, than by raising the oxygen pressure. What does happen in acclimatization is that inactive capillaries open, thus decreasing the distance oxygen must diffuse from blood to cells. As we picture it today, the process of acclimatization to high altitude occurs mainly in ventilation, circulation, and oxygen transport. These changes set in motion cellular changes which, ultimately, make acclimatization possible.

8. MOUNTAIN SICKNESS

Edward Whymper, the most famous climber in the Victorian era, in 1876 described his experience with mountain sickness dramatically:

> I found myself flat on my back . . . incapable of making even the least exertion . . . we were experiencing our first attack of mountain sickness. . . . We were feverish, had intense headache and were unable to satisfy our desire for air. . . . Headache for all three of us was intense and rendered us almost frantic or crazy.

A famous contemporary, Edward FitzGerald, was equally vivid:

> I was only able to advance one or two steps at a time and then I had to stop, panting for breath, my struggles alternating with violent fits of nausea. At times I would fall down, and each time had greater difficulty rising; black specks swam across my sight; I was like one walking in a dream, so dizzy and sick that the whole mountain seemed whirling about me. . . . As I got lower . . . I improved.

The first complete description of the various forms of altitude illness was written in 1913 by Thomas Ravenhill, doctor to a mining camp in the Andes. Though he thought them distinct entities and gave them different names and assigned different causes, there is no mistaking the clinical picture. He knew more about altitude illnesses than anyone else. His paper was published in an obscure journal and found only recently. Ravenhill was wounded in World War I and was unable to pursue his pioneering work, but this one paper assures him standing among the pioneers.

The Problem

Because we consider altitude illnesses a *collection* of signs and symptoms rather than several discrete afflictions, I will discuss them as a continuum or a spectrum of a single problem—hypoxia—sharing many signs and symptoms.[1]

Different people under similar conditions sometimes respond quite differently to altitude; we know little about why. For most people, at least four factors determine whether one will be sick or well after going to altitude: First, the speed of ascent; the slower the climb the fewer the symptoms. Second, the altitude reached; the higher one goes the more likely are problems. Third, one's health at the time; malnutrition, dehydration, fatigue, and any of several illnesses will increase the risk. Finally, individual characteristics, genetic influences, or some unusual metabolic or circulatory variant, all may affect susceptibility.

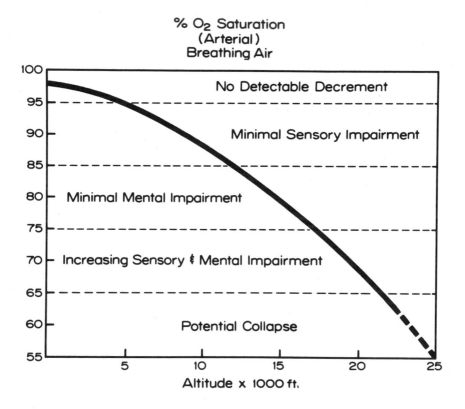

Figure 8-1

[1]Symptoms are what the patient feels; signs are what the observer sees or hears, though often the patient does not.

Acute Mountain Sickness

Recently a survey of thirty-nine hundred visitors to a Colorado mountain resort showed that 24 percent of those who had gone rapidly from sea level to 3,000 meters (10,000 feet) experienced three or more of the symptoms of AMS. Usually the symptoms subsided in a day or two and only rarely progressed to a more serious form. One third of those with AMS said they had limited their activities as a result. If we assume that these sick people did not spend some of the money they might otherwise have spent for food or drink or sport, the loss of revenue for resort owners is very substantial, due to a preventable, avoidable illness. And this does not include the human suffering, occasional deaths, or the visitors who leave early and never return. Smaller studies have collected comparable data at other elevations.

The impact of altitude is determined by the priority the body places on oxygen supply to each organ system. The brain ranks high: it receives about 15 percent of the blood pumped by the heart and uses over 20 percent of all the oxygen consumed; the cerebral cortex (where complex mental activity occurs), is the most demanding. It should not be surprising, then, that hypoxia affects the higher centers of the brain early and that judgment and high intellectual functions are the first to suffer. If you have ever arrived late at a cocktail party, you may have observed that the guests aren't as witty or alert as they think they are, and often don't realize how impaired they may be. The effects of hypoxia are much like those of alcohol. It is probable that many tragedies on very high mountains have been due at least in part to poor judgment caused by lack of oxygen.

Why headache is such a prominent symptom of mountain sickness is unclear. Brain tissue does not have nerve endings that feel pain, but the filmy membranes that cover it and its blood vessels are very sensitive. To protect the brain when its blood supply contains too little oxygen, sensors increase its blood flow, so the distended vessels or engorged brain tissue pressing on the membranes may be the cause of headache. But blood flow to the brain is *decreased* as lack of oxygen stimulates breathing, washing carbon dioxide out of lungs and blood. Consequently, whether brain blood flow increases or decreases will depend on the balance between hypoxia and hypocapnia and on the sensitivity of the receptors that allocate blood flow. This could explain why the severity of altitude headache differs among individuals, and why different studies of cerebral blood flow at altitude often produce contradictory results. Direct measurements of pressure in the brain (as reflected in the cerebrospinal fluid which bathes it) have been contradictory. A small recent study suggested that the pressure within the skull is not related to the headache, but some other studies show the opposite. Much more work needs to be done.

Nausea, vomiting, and disturbed sleep, so typical of mountain sickness, may be due to swelling or to altered blood flow to the midbrain where the centers that control these functions are located.

A bad attack of AMS is not trivial, and it has notable but reversible effects on physiology. It is known that fluid leaks from the circulating blood into tissues, concentrating the blood, and causing an apparent increase in the red cell count. This begins almost immediately after arrival, and for some people causes puffiness (edema) of face, hands, and feet. Many people do not develop edema because their kidneys compensate for the fluid shift by putting out more urine. German doctors called this *hohen-diuresen,* and we consider it a favorable response. The blood is thickened, true, but those who respond this way don't develop edema, and by drinking a lot of extra water, the hemoconcentration is corrected.

Contrariwise, those who develop edema do not pass as much urine, and do have more symptoms. It has been shown that such people secrete more of a hormone which inhibits urine formation, the antidiuretic hormone or ADH, formed by the pituitary gland.

In the high mountain environment, cold, physical activity, shortage of food and water, fatigue, and fear, all confound the fluid and electrolyte responses to hypoxia. These co-existing factors may explain the contradictory reports that hypoxia stimulates, has no effect, or inhibits release of hormones like ADH or renin precursors and stimulates or inhibits aldosterone release. We have already seen that both rate and depth of breathing increase very soon after arrival at altitude, and pulse rate and cardiac stroke volume also increase in most people. Blood pressure goes up, though a bit later, and not in all individuals. These are healthy, normal compensations that seem designed to sustain a near normal amount of oxygen entering blood and being transported to the needy cells. They are not evidence of AMS.

Other responses are also occurring in the first hours and days after arrival at altitude. The adrenal glands produce more than thirty hormones, some of which are important in hypoxia. From the cortex (the outside) of the adrenals come aldosterone, the glucocorticoids, and the mineralocorticoids, all of which have powerful effects on carbohydrates and on salt and water balance. From the medulla (center) of the glands come the crucially important hormones epinephrine (commonly called adrenaline) and its analog nor-epinephrine. The secretion of these is stimulated by the sympathetic nervous system, which in turn is affected by stress—any kind of stress.

Other hormones from the adrenal glands (and one called atrial natriurretic peptide or ANP because it is secreted in a small area within the atrium of the heart) are also important. We know a great deal about the individual hormones and their actions, but their interactions are so complex that we don't understand fully their net effect on humans at altitude. Indeed this varies from person to person and circumstance to circumstance.

One attractive hypothesis which has not been proven, and is disputed by some, is based on the dynamic equilibrium between ions on each side of the cell membranes in all parts of the body. What is called the "sodium pump" is a bioelectric activity that maintains normal concentrations inside and outside each cell, even pumping ions through the cell walls against higher concentration. This is an energy-intensive process and requires a great deal of oxygen. The theory runs that lack of oxygen causes the pump to falter, allowing water to accumulate within the cells as sodium leaks out.

From this brief summary we can see that the immediate responses to altitude, and to moderate hypoxia from other causes as well, cause reversible changes in physiology or function rather than lasting damage. Only when the hypoxia is very severe or very rapid do we find death and destruction of body tissues. Humans are able to tolerate mild oxygen lack by making these and other changes, as we will see in chapter 9 when we discuss acclimatization.

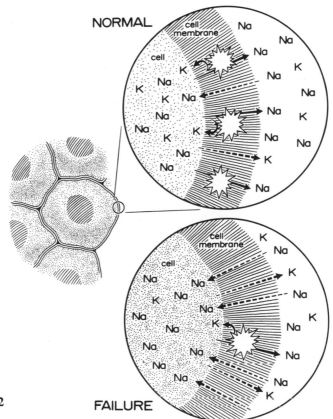

Figure 8-2

High Altitude Pulmonary Edema

HAPE is less frequent but more serious than AMS, and, like AMS, is far from new. Fifteen hundred years ago, a Chinese archivist, Hui Jiao, wrote a dramatic account:

> The wind was chilling to the bones on the shady north side of the Lesser Snowy Mountains. Hui Jing was in a serious condition, frothing at the mouth, losing his strength rapidly and fainting away now and then. Finally he dropped dead on the snowy ground, although Fa Hsien and Dao Zheng had tried their best to save him.

Several studies have shown that most people going to even moderate altitudes develop fluid in the thin, loose lung tissue that separates alveoli from the capillaries. Usually this is promptly reabsorbed. If it is not, but accumulates within the alveoli, passage of oxygen from lung to blood is impaired, the alveolar-arterial gradient or pressure drop increases, hypoxia worsens, more fluid leaks into the air sacs, and the victim literally drowns in his own juices.

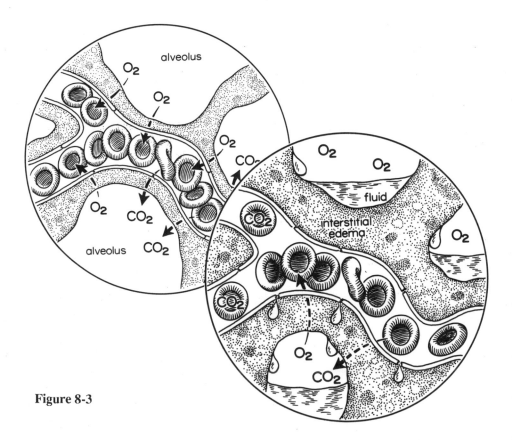

Figure 8-3

The symptoms of HAPE are increasing shortness of breath, even while resting, and an irritative cough that soon produces a frothy, often blood-tinged sputum. Mental confusion, extreme fatigue, and a staggering drunken walk may follow soon; the patient will slip into coma unless treated promptly.In contrast to AMS, there are many signs indicating the presence of HAPE. The victim looks anxious, is restless, and usually has a rapid, bounding pulse, and quick, shallow breathing. Cyanosis (the bluish tint to lips and nails that heralds less well-oxygenated blood) is a bad sign. The cough is irritating, and after a while produces copious sputum, often pink, and sometimes bloody. There may be a slight fever which is alarming. The white blood cell count may be increased. More fever and a higher white cell count suggest an infection masquerading as HAPE.The chest X-ray is typical, and not easily mistaken for anything else.

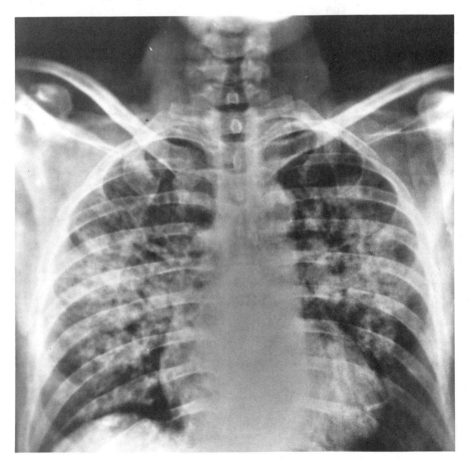

Figure 8-4

The heart shadow is normal, or, rarely, slightly enlarged. Throughout the lungs, mostly on the right side, one sees areas where the X-ray penetrates less well. These shadows, often described as fluffy, represent accumulations of fluid, and they are usually seen toward the outer sections of the lungs rather than close to the middle as is the case in heart failure. The X-ray picture is very different from pneumonia, or tumor, or any inflammatory process. Surprisingly, the X-ray changes do not exactly parallel the physical signs: one can see a bad-looking X-ray in a patient who is not very sick and has only a few crackling sounds called rales, and the opposite is also true.

Sounds heard in the lungs vary a great deal. In quite a few people with AMS one can hear scratchy sounds, called *rales,* here and there in the lungs. These are probably due to a bit of fluid in the loose interstitial lung tissue. In early cases of HAPE, there may be very little to hear, but soon squeaks, groans, and rattles can be heard, together with more rales, in many parts of the lungs. In its early stages, HAPE is often mistaken for flu or a chest cold, but HAPE can progress with deadly speed to a life-threatening illness, far more dangerous than pneumonia:

> J was an experienced airline pilot and strong athlete. He and his wife drove to a mountain resort where they began skiing soon after arrival. On the second day J complained of headache and weakness; he had more trouble breathing than his friends did, and by afternoon he was falling a lot. His wife urged him to go down and to see a doctor. Instead he went directly to their hotel where they later found him asleep. Before dawn next morning his severe cough and struggles to breathe wakened his wife. Friends carried him to a car and to a doctor, but his heart stopped; he was resuscitated, treated for HAPE, and flown to hospital. He died eleven days later with extensive brain damage.

This sad outcome was the result of untreated AMS progressing to HAPE and causing cardiac arrest, brain damage, and death. J had ample warning that something was terribly wrong; his judgment led him astray, and neither he nor his wife and friends realized until too late how seriously ill he was.

During the past fifty years, as more and more people began to go to high mountains and resorts more rapidly and easily, similar tragedies have occurred hundreds of times. Altitude illnesses occur and can be fatal, not only on the high Himalayas, or Andes, or the Rockies, but also anywhere above 2,400 meters (8,000 feet), wherever people go up too fast.

Because HAPE can be so serious, even though not common, it has attracted more interest, study, and speculation than the milder AMS, with which it is intertwined. Consequently we have learned a great deal about HAPE in the last few years because it frequently strikes the young, the strong, and the brave so tragically. HAPE is a condition in which disordered function progresses, often swiftly, to structural damage to the target organ—the lungs. How does this happen? Here is what we know, or think we know today.

The small arterioles of the lungs are peculiarly sensitive to lack of oxygen, which causes them to contract (a vasoconstrictor response). This increases blood pressure in the arterial side of the pulmonary circulation. From the normal 12 to 20 torr, pressure in the pulmonary arteries increases to 30 or 50 torr, or even higher, and is further increased by exertion. This elevated pressure stimulates release of many powerful substances, whether directly because of pressure within the vessels, or indirectly due to shearing forces along their lining. We call these "biologically active substances" because they are neither exactly hormones nor enzymes but transients. Their family tree is only partly known. What is important about these substances, which seem to occur mostly in the lung, is that some of them increase, while others decrease, reactions of blood and blood vessels. For example, some cause blood platelets to stick together more readily, while others decrease such clumping. Some increase the muscular tone of the small arteries in the lung, and thereby maintain high pressure. Others relax this vasoconstriction. Some increase the leakiness (permeability) of small vessels. Many of them are very short-lived and thus hard to detect, but others persist and can be assayed in blood and even in urine. Just what influence they have outside of the lungs is not clear at this time. But the effect they have on the lungs is critically important in HAPE.

Several years ago Peter Hackett and Robert Schoene and their colleagues on Denali (Mount McKinley, 6,096 meters; 20,320 feet) studied the nature of the fluid that fills the lungs of patients with HAPE. By passing a flexible tube (bronchoscope) deep into the lungs, they were able to suck out some of the fluid for analysis. They found that the fluid contained a lot of protein and a number of megakaryocytes (scavenger blood cells). The fluid also was rich in the various members of the eicosanoid family. This is what one might expect if the barrier between the blood stream and the air sac has begun to leak. It is not typical of an infection or inflammation.

At this point the evidence pointed to a high pressure, high permeability situation as the cause of HAPE. There were still uncertainties: Were the eicosanoids a cause or a result of this leak? And how did the large red blood cells reach the alveoli? Something in addition to a membrane leak seemed likely. We have speculated for several years that when the delicate lining of the capillaries in the lung stretches under the increased pressure, the normally tight junctions between the lining cells might open up. These tiny openings would increase the leakiness and might even allow red blood cells to pass from the capillaries into the alveoli, thus explaining the blood-tinged sputum.

But we could not be certain the pressure was transmitted from the muscular, constricted arterioles to the small capillaries. One rarely has there been an opportunity to examine immediately the lungs of someone who has just died of HAPE, and therefore it has been difficult to determine whether or not these tight junctions had opened to produce holes. West and colleagues have demonstrated that these tight junctions do open in rabbits when pulmonary artery pressure is increased, but this does not explain why most people with high pulmonary artery pressure do not develop HAPE.

Another theory, advanced thirty years ago, has surfaced again. It had been known for many years that certain head injuries and other rarer brain disorders sometimes cause pulmonary edema, and a high permeability, high pressure edema at that. Based on elaborate animal studies, Gerald Moss believed he could produce typical HAPE by transfusing the brain with hypoxic blood while the lung was supplied with well-oxygenated blood. He suggested that HAPE might be due to lack of oxygen in the brain. No one has yet repeated this work, though there are some promising developments.

For many years Herbert Hultgren, arguably the leading authority on HAPE, has believed in a different theory. Noting that the X-ray picture of HAPE is very different from other lung disorders, Hultgren theorized that the fluffy patches seen on X-rays are areas of edema where there is too much blood and not enough air. We talk of "perfusion"—areas with good blood flow—and "ventilation"—areas with adequate air flow—and Hultgren argues that when there is a disparity between the two—called "ventilation-perfusion inequity"—edema results.

Two clinical conditions support this opinion. The first is a rare congenital condition in which one lung does not develop its normal pulmonary artery, receiving blood from many small vessels instead. A score of patients with this abnormality have developed typical HAPE in the normal lung at very low altitudes—even as low as 1,500 meters (5,000 feet). Hultgren's hypothesis would hold that the normal lung was over-perfused by the increased blood flow and pressure due to even mild hypoxia.

The second condition is one which follows pulmonary embolism, the passage of blood clots from leg or other veins into the lungs, where they block smaller vessels. If there are enough of such small clots, or a few larger ones, typical areas of ventilation-perfusion inequity result, and these patients develop pulmonary edema in the affected lung. There are suggestions that people who have residual small obstructions from embolism in the past may be at risk for HAPE when they go to altitude, but this needs verification.

Many aspects of HAPE need much further study. First is the fact that a few individuals have repeated episodes of HAPE. In fact, they tend to develop HAPE whenever they go to even moderate altitude. They are perfectly healthy and often excellent athletes or experienced mountaineers. Extensive studies have not explained why. Some, but not all of them, develop much higher pulmonary artery blood pressure than do other people when at altitude. Some, but not all, have a sluggish respiratory response to oxygen lack (what is called a blunted hypoxic ventilatory response.) We can only speculate that their biologically active substances differ in kind or potency from normal.

Second is the curious fact that some, but not all, people who live at altitude occasionally develop HAPE when they return after a short stay near sea level. This is called re-entry HAPE. Though little statistically indisputable data prove this, the anecdotal evidence can no longer be denied. We do not understand why this may happen.

Then there is strong anecdotal evidence that an apparently minor respiratory infection—a simple cold, or a mild virus—seems to increase the risk of HAPE. Again, we do not have statistical proof, but the evidence is persuasive. Whether there is a real difference between men and women, or between adults and children, remains to be shown. We can not even say for certain whether older people are at greater risk. So far the data only suggest that HAPE is more common at younger age. Of one thing we are quite sure: HAPE is a disturbance of the lungs and not due to heart failure as Ravenhill and others believed until 1960. Furthermore, for HAPE to develop, not only must pulmonary artery pressure be high, but membrane permeability must also be increased. We know this because almost everyone has high pulmonary artery pressure at altitude, but few develop HAPE. Also, some people develop high pulmonary artery pressure (pulmonary hypertension) at sea level but do not develop edema for many years if ever, and when they do, it is different from HAPE. However, to confuse the matter, some patients with HAPE improve very quickly when pulmonary artery pressure is rapidly lowered by medication.

High Altitude Cerebral Edema

When the central nervous system is most affected at altitude, we use the term HACE to describe a much less common illness, on the assumption that parts of the brain have become waterlogged. The signs and symptoms are often dramatic and frightening.

A strong Japanese mountaineer climbed rapidly to 19,000 feet on Mount Logan, where he became confused and unable to walk. His companions carried him down a few thousand feet, and he was flown to low altitude. He remained irrational and hallucinating for a day, and unable to stand, or to use his hands or fingers for two additional days. Later he made a complete recovery after returning home.

A language barrier made it difficult to assess symptoms in this man, but he was lucky to have been evacuated so rapidly. Had he remained longer at altitude, he might have died, or been left with permanent brain damage.

A young paratrooper was flown to 17,500 feet. Though he did not mention any symptoms such as headache, he became confused, and sixteen hours after arrival became comatose. During a midnight evacuation by air he seemed near death, but he regained consciousness eight hours after reaching low altitude and treatment. He too made a complete recovery.

These two cases suggest that the brain may be severely affected without any other indication of altitude illness, but they are unusual. Far more frequently, the victim has other evidence of AMS or of HAPE, although the signs of HACE may dominate.

A middle-aged man visited a doctor two days after arrival at a ski resort; he complained of headache, nausea, inability to sleep and was told he had mountain sickness. Next day he returned, short of breath, confused, and walking clumsily. His AMS had progressed to HACE. He went down to lower altitude, recovering en route.

One early warning of HACE (and also of HAPE) is difficulty with walking, or, less often, with finger and hand motions. The individual tends to stagger, has trouble with balance, and soon is unable to walk a straight line or to stand steadily with feet together and eyes closed. He walks as if drunk! This may be the only evidence that something is wrong. More often the person is a little confused, and, though tending to conceal the fact, may hear voices or see things that aren't really there. These hallucinations can seem very real:

An able medical doctor wrote me a long description of hearing voices and seeing strangers at 4,200 meters (14,000 feet) during a climb. He had enough sense to recognize the danger and to go down, where he quickly recovered. Several years later, at an even higher altitude, he again hallucinated but did not recognize this. He became violent; his companions tape-recorded his protests and were able to get him down. Later he denied the whole affair.

The term HACE may be misleading because we do not know for sure that there is edema in the brain, except in severe, fatal cases where autopsy has shown a waterlogged brain. What we do see is disturbance in function, as if some nerve pathways were short-circuited or misconnected. Alcohol causes the same kind of temporary disruption, and once again we are reminded of some similarity between hypoxia and intoxication.

More often than not victims with AMS or HAPE also show some evidence of HACE. They are a little unsteady, a bit confused, not quite right. Toshio

Kobayashi obtained computerized scans of the brain in patients with severe HAPE and found that there was some evidence of edema in parts of the brain. In severe cases of either HAPE or HACE the pressure of cerebrospinal fluid (clear liquid which bathes the brain) is increased, presumably due to edema.

Although there are still too many deaths from altitude illnesses, only a few cases diagnosed as HACE have been autopsied. In these the brain is heavy with edema and contains many small, and often some larger, hemorrhages. These small bleeding areas raise important questions: Are they due to HACE? Did they occur only in the agonal stage? Do they indicate other internal bleeding similar to the tiny splinter hemorrhages we see in the eyes and beneath fingernails and rarely in the kidney? If these tiny hemorrhages also occur in the brain at very high altitude, may they leave lasting damage to the brain, our most vulnerable tissue?

The latter remains a nagging question. Climbers breathing only the thin air about them have reached all the highest summits. Have their brains been permanently damaged by hypoxia? Some respected physician-mountaineers believe such exposure does leave some damage. Others point to the hundreds of high summiters who have lived to a ripe and bright old age. Few studies have compared neurological examinations before with those made after a major expedition, but one of these showed a small change—decreased speed of finger-tapping—one year later. Quite a few mountaineers who have gone very high have come home to depression, divorce, or difficulty settling into the daily round. We need other, more conclusive evidence.

Obviously, collecting this kind of subtle information is very difficult and requires a careful examination before and after the subjects have been on a major expedition. One study of intellectual function is not very persuasive. In another controlled study, two similar groups were compared, one with and one without altitude exposure. No difference was found.

A healthy twenty-five-year-old man acclimatized well, taking twenty days to reach 18,500 feet where he felt perfectly well and strong. Next morning, (as he said later), "nothing worked very well." He had difficulty thinking and talking, and had to be helped off the mountain, developing a high fever en route. He became unconscious during helicopter evacuation and spent months in a hospital slowly regaining partial use of his arms and legs. Many years later he is still permanently brain damaged.

A forty-five-year-old doctor was high on Everest, felt strong and well, but suddenly became partially paralyzed. He managed to get down to base camp where he became temporarily blind. The weakness in his arm and leg slowly improved. Careful studies later resulted in a diagnosis of stroke due to a blood clot or a small hemorrhage in the brain. He recovered, returned several times to high altitude, but still has slight changes in speech and some fine motions.

The first patient is believed to have had a serious infection of his brain (perhaps encephalitis), rather than damage from hypoxia. The problem experienced by the second could be explained by a stroke, an accident that can happen anywhere, anytime to older individuals. Still, both raise troublesome questions.

A famous climber has gone very high repeatedly in the last thirty years. Recently he has developed HAPE or HACE, or some major problem, each time at a somewhat lower altitude. Now in his sixties, he does not show any more change than would be expected from aging alone.

A psychiatrist studied more than forty men who had gone very high once or several times. He found persistent emotional problems in many. But several of the group had experienced psychiatric problems before going to altitude, several had had earlier head injuries, or had been extremely sick while on the mountain. He is a conscientious physician, and his observations cannot be ignored, even though most of the cases are distorted by more than hypoxia.

What can we conclude? Not much for certain! Those who would ban climbing without extra oxygen above 7,500 meters (25,000 feet) are unreasonable. Yet those who deliberately spend many days at extreme altitude, exposed to many stresses like cold, hunger, and dehydration in addition to hypoxia, should realize that they may be risking permanent damage.

At this time, my own belief is that hypoxia alone rarely leaves a permanent scar in the brain, unless—and this is an important reservation—the exposure is for many days, and combined with other extreme stresses.

Having said this, remember that people who have a cardiac arrest, or sudden severe obstruction to breathing, at sea level will probably suffer lasting brain damage if the severe hypoxia lasts more than four or five minutes.

Less clear are the emotional and intellectual changes we see in older people (and a few young ones too) who have chronic lung disease that keeps them moderately hypoxic all the time. Their intellectual powers often seem subtly impaired, and their brains may be damaged, but it is not possible to tell how much of this is due to natural aging.

Chronic Mountain Sickness

Three more conditions must be described because of what they may teach us about certain sea level problems. The first, Chronic Mountain Sickness

(CMS), is often called Monge's disease after the man who first described it in the Andes in 1928, Carlos Monge pére. CMS occurs only in long-time residents at altitudes over 3,300 meters (11,000 feet). Though a few cases have been reported from the high regions in Central Asia, CMS occurs most frequently among those who live high in the Andes.

The signs and symptoms are striking. Gradually, over months, the victim (usually male) develops a flushed, purplish color, becomes weak, and has many vague aches and pains, especially in the chest. He cannot concentrate, becomes irritable, and may even hallucinate. He is short of breath even at rest, tires easily, develops swelling in the face and legs, and often forms blood clots in his veins. His blood is dark reddish and thicker than normal. Red cells may increase from a normal of around 4.5 million to as much as 7-8 million, and occupy 75 percent of the blood volume (as shown in the hematocrit). Pulmonary artery pressure is high, and sometimes the systemic blood pressure is also abnormal. Soon his heart enlarges, and, unless treated, he develops congestive heart failure and will die.

If the patient goes to sea level, the condition slowly improves, and unless too far advanced, disappears, but it will return months after he returns to altitude. Phlebotomy (removing blood), or reducing the number of red blood cells with medication, temporarily relieves but does not cure the illness. CMS is an exaggeration of the normal adaptation to altitude, which we know as acclimatization, but we do not understand why this happens.

CMS is of special interest because it resembles an affliction that is being recognized more and more often at sea level, although it is considered a collection of problems rather than a single entity. One of these used to be called "Pickwickian syndrome" because the victims were fat, always sleepy, tired or considered lazy, and short of breath. Today we use the less picturesque term "alveolar hypoventilation" because the problem is due to poor exchange of air deep in the lungs. What this does is to keep the individual short of oxygen all the time, as if living at altitude, and some develop a condition similar to CMS.

Sleep Apnea

Another condition is probably more common, in a mild form, than we realize. Known as "sleep apnea," it is due to irregular breathing during sleep, with complete stoppage for thirty or forty seconds every few minutes. During and after these periods of absent breathing, the blood oxygen falls sharply. The periods of apnea can occupy a large part of the night, and therefore the patient is in effect sleeping at altitude, sometimes very high. Because the apnea often rouses him, sleep is interrupted, and he is sleepy all day. Several men with sleep apnea have had automobile accidents because they fell asleep at the wheel. Like CMS, it is much more frequent in men.

Sleep apnea may originate in the brain, or it may be due to a common problem—snoring. In this case it is commonly called "intermittent upper airway obstruction" (IUAO) to distinguish it from still another problem, obstruction in the *lower* airways. This latter is more common, and better known as "chronic obstructive pulmonary disease" (COPD), a term that includes emphysema, chronic bronchitis, and other abnormalities too many to discuss here.

Subacute Mountain Sickness

A third unusual condition was first described by Menon after the Indo-Chinese border conflict in 1962. The Chinese troops had been well acclimatized by months at altitude, but the Indian soldiers were rushed up to 3,600 meters (12,000 feet) and stayed there for weeks or months. A large number had to be immediately evacuated with HAPE and HACE, but some others were taken down after many weeks because of what is now called "subacute mountain sickness." More cases have recently occurred among Pakistani troops stationed very high in the Karakoram Himalaya for many weeks.

The same condition has also been described in Han Chinese children taken from the lowlands to high Tibet. Little seems to be gained by considering it to be different from the adult form. Both are variants of chronic mountain sickness, and, like CMS, are due to heart failure resulting from pulmonary hypertension.

Subacute mountain sickness is quite similar to a problem which develops in certain strains of cattle—brisket disease—when they are taken from low to moderate altitude. Like cattle with this disease, men with subacute mountain sickness develop an enlarged heart (principally the right ventricle) because of their high pulmonary artery pressure. Then as the heart fails, edema accumulates in the legs, liver, both lungs, and (in cattle) the brisket. This altitude problem is due to heart failure.

High Altitude Retinal Hemorrhage

Twenty-five years ago on Mount Logan, our group noticed some tiny hemorrhages in the back of the eyes (the retina) of a few of the young people working in the laboratory at 5,250 meters (17,500 feet). These little bleeding spots did not cause any symptoms, and the climbers were unaware of them. After our reports were published, other scientists saw the hemorrhages—named High Altitude Retinal Hemorrhages (HARH) in many mountaineers—even as low as 3,000 meters (10,000 feet). They are quite common, rarely cause symptoms or leave scars, disappear within a few days even at altitude, and do not appear to be related to other altitude illnesses, to exertion, or to length of stay at altitude. A few similar splinter hemorrhages under the fingernails have been described. Nosebleeds were very common on mountains many years ago, but we do not hear much about them today.

The reason HARH have attracted notice is the serious question of whether or not they indicate bleeding elsewhere—in the brain for instance. As we saw earlier, this is an important question. Some people do develop abnormalities in the blood clotting mechanisms at altitude, but here again there is much individual variation and many unanswered questions.

Prevention

For most people, most of the time, altitude illness can be avoided by taking time to go to altitude: give your body a chance to adjust naturally. We have become a medicated society, however, and many people want a magic pill against everything. If you can't or won't take time, then protective medications are available. One of these, Diamox (acetazolamide), has been effectively used to prevent AMS for more than thirty years. It seems to prevent HAPE and HACE as well, although it is almost impossible to prove this because these two conditions are not very common.

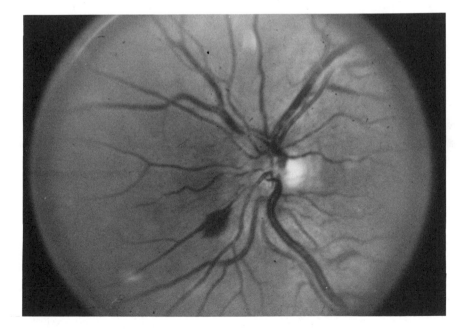

Figure 8-5

Diamox inhibits an enzyme, carbonic anhydrase, that occurs in almost all tissues. This powerful enzyme affects the reversible reaction between carbon dioxide and water. The simplest explanation of the benefits of Diamox is that it enables the body to blow off more carbon dioxide, while decreasing the alkalosis that results. This means better alveolar ventilation and higher alveolar oxygen pressure. By inhibiting carbonic anhydrase, Diamox enables the kidney to excrete more bicarbonate, which enhances acclimatization. It is usually only a mild diuretic, but for some people Diamox does stimulate a really brisk flow of urine.

Diamox is effective for most lowlanders going to moderate altitude, and perhaps for altitude residents returning after a short stay at low altitude. It has been called an artificial acclimatizer because it strengthens or hastens the natural processes of overbreathing, excretion of bicarbonate, and stabilization of blood pH. Many people taking Diamox notice tingling in the fingers and toes or around the mouth. This is related to the size of the dose and is not a true side effect. Occasionally Diamox causes dizziness, and weakness. People who are sensitive to sun sometimes develop a skin reaction similar to that which may result from sulfa drugs, to which Diamox is distantly related.

Just how much Diamox to take, and when to take it, is still debated. For many years most doctors recommended one 250 mg tablet twice a day for two or three days before ascent and for several days afterwards. However, since the effect of this enzyme-inhibitor wears off in eight or ten hours, such a dosage schedule seems excessive. Some evidence suggests that this large dose (which is normal for other purposes) can cause muscle weakness while it is taken.

Experience now suggests that a half tablet (125 mg) on the morning and evening of ascent, and twice a day for two more days, is enough to protect without causing the unpleasant tingling and without spoiling the taste of beer and other carbonated drinks. This leaves open the possibility of adding more of the medication to treat symptoms if they occur.

The steroid dexamethasone has also been used for preventing AMS. Four mg taken by mouth before starting up to an altitude where you anticipate AMS is effective for many people. It is not without slight risk, and it is not the preventive of choice. Some experienced climbing doctors point out that the slight euphoria from dexamethasone may hide warning symptoms, and, when dexamethasone is stopped, serious HAPE or HACE may suddenly develop.

Another medicine, nifedipine, is being used, especially by those who are unusually susceptible to HAPE. Since the effects of this calcium channel blocker wear off in a few hours, the slowly absorbed preparation, or even the dermal patch would seem better than the oral dose. However, calcium blockers affect all the small arteries in the body and can lower blood pressure too far and too rapidly for safety. It is likely that using nifedipine as a preventive will be limited to unusual individuals at special risk.

Forty years ago two other preventives were tried: ammonium chloride and methylene blue. The latter was reported to be effective in two studies and should be restudied using modern methods.

Still, the best prevention is to let our natural defenses work. Again, take time to go high. Drink extra water to prevent dehydration—even though this has not been proven to be an effective preventive. Don't add the effect of alcohol to that of hypoxia. Eat lightly for a few days. Don't overexert yourself until you have adjusted to less oxygen. Listen to your body!

Treatment

People with mild AMS or HAPE usually improve even at altitude after a few days of rest and can then continue with what they came to do. Providing the condition does not become worse, and if the patient can be carefully watched, a day or two of rest at altitude may be sufficient.

All forms of altitude illness are improved simply by going down a few thousand feet. If HACE is suspected, early descent is wise because this is more subtle and more serious than AMS. The next best step after descent is breathing additional oxygen in order to raise the inspired oxygen pressure to that at sea level. Both of these steps relieve the headache rapidly and completely and make breathing easier. Mental confusion also clears, but more slowly (just as after too much alcohol). Both descent and oxygen are easy and logical, and they work.

Many anecdotes and a few studies indicate that Diamox will relieve the symptoms of AMS, sometimes dramatically. It is a simple and inexpensive remedy for symptoms, which can be unpleasant though rarely serious. Does Diamox work as well for HAPE? A few field experiences suggest that it does, though it does not appear to be as effective as the calcium blocker nifedipine.

No Diamox dosage for treatment has been established, but one 250 mg tablet should be tried, followed in four or five hours by another. Except for the cautions mentioned above, Diamox is quite safe and sometimes remarkably helpful.

Another treatment is to place the patient in an environment of increased pressure. This can be done best by placing the patient in a bag or tent made of tough fabric that can be sealed tightly and inflated to a few pounds more pressure than the outside environment. The pressurized bag is as effective as breathing oxygen or going down several thousand feet. There are several sizes and shapes of bags, the best-known in the United States being the Gamow Tent. Though not suitable for use over more than a few hours, one may save a life when neither descent nor oxygen are available options.

Ways to eliminate excess fluid, especially the edema in the lungs, seem logical, and many years ago, strong diuretics were used. They were soon found to carry a serious risk of decreasing blood volume too much, thereby converting a person with HAPE who could still walk into a litter case. Diuretics simply pull water from the blood, concentrating it even further, and are likely to make the problem worse, not better. Only under certain desperate circumstances, when nothing else is available, might a strong diuretic save a life threatened by HAPE.

9. STAYING WELL AT ALTITUDE

Even though adventurers, explorers, and travellers were few and slow to go to high places, throughout the centuries many generations have lived there. On thirty-five Andean summits there remain traces of ancient habitations, some of them as high as 6,600 meters (22,000 feet), and some of them obviously small hamlets. These stone houses, shrines, piles of wood, and other relics strongly suggest that five hundred years ago Andean people worked and worshipped on higher places than anyone lives today. We do not know how long they were there, but if not permanently, at least they stayed for long periods. Even including the high Tibetan plateau we know of no permanent habitations above 5,100 meters (17,000 feet) anywhere in the world today. A few caretakers live for periods of several years at a mine at 6,000 meters (20,000 feet) in the Andes, but they frequently descend for vacation at a more hospitable elevation.

Some scientists today have teased us by suggesting that people are more nearly "normal" at moderate altitude, say a mile above sea level, but anemic and less effective at sea level. The weight of evidence, however, shows that above 1,500 meters (5,000 feet) humans do not function quite as well, even after years, as do their cohorts near sea level. The deficits are subtle, very subtle, and hotly denied by many, but they can be demonstrated. Above 3,500 meters (11,500 feet) permanent residents have a decreased work capacity compared to sea level residents, though they can do more than can recent visitors to altitude.

At 5,400 meters (18,000 feet) man has reached his ceiling if he stays for more than a few weeks; above this he is clearly impaired. As I shall describe, only a marvelous series of integrated adjustments make it possible for a few strong-willed men and women, apparently little different from you and me, to climb to the highest point on earth where there is only a third of the oxygen available at sea level. This mechanism is called acclimatization, and remarkably, people who are ill with a number of medical problems that affect their oxygen supply at sea level adjust in many ways like the healthy acclimatizing mountaineer. (CHAP 9)

If so many people are made ill by altitude, and some strong and healthy people die, even at 3,000 meters (10,000 feet), how is it that hundreds have survived for weeks on very high mountains, even summiting Everest without supplementary oxygen? Are these supermen and women? How are they different from the rank and file?

Any sea level person, taken abruptly to 6,000 to 7,000 meters (20,000 feet), will be almost incapacitated in less than half an hour, and death will not be far. At 8,700 meters (29,000 feet), where less than a third of the oxygen to which we are accustomed is available, tragic examples have shown how quickly sea level humans die.

The process that protects the mountaineer is most accurately called acclimatization. We define this as "a series of changes throughout the body which tend to restore the oxygen pressure in the tissues toward that at sea level." The words are carefully chosen: at high altitude the oxygen supply only *tends* to approach *toward* normal; cells remain oxygen-hungry on top of Everest. No human is normal there. Most are not far from death. The integrated process of acclimatization takes time, and to climb the last few thousand feet on Mount Everest, adjustment must be more rapid. But in fact, little improvement occurs at that extreme altitude, and the summiter must climb the last thousands of feet relying on his courage, determination, and drive rather than on more acclimatization than the degree that enabled him to get that far.

When we go to the mountains, at first the body struggles to maintain its status quo. Normal processes are exaggerated in the effort to sustain a normal oxygen supply to our cells. Ventilation increases enormously: "It took me six breaths to take one step upward," said one climber. This rushing tide of air raises the alveolar oxygen by bringing fresh air deeper into the lungs. But it also removes carbon dioxide and lowers alveolar carbon dioxide dangerously, and the blood becomes more alkaline. Chris Pizzo, who collected the only samples of alveolar air yet obtained on the top of Everest, says he was breathing about ninety times a minute there.

Even at much lower altitudes, the new arrival is aware of increased breathing. Also, in order to carry more oxygen more rapidly to the starving cells, the heart beats harder and faster, pumping several times its normal volume per minute. Small capillaries, some of which are usually not open at sea level and at rest, are recruited to provide better blood flow to tissues. Shortly after reaching altitude, blood volume decreases because plasma leaks out of the capillaries into the tissues and as a result the circulating blood appears to contain more hemoglobin per unit volume than it did at sea level. In reality, the body has almost the same amount of circulating hemoglobin and the same oxygen capacity. This is not completely accurate, because some reserve blood may be squeezed from the spleen into active service, as it is in race horses. The nervous system is alerted to the lack of oxygen and signals many organs to respond, some rapidly, some more gradually, by release of hormones to activate more sustainable responses.

These "struggle responses" are the most effective, best-known, and most studied immediate reactions to hypoxia. They are soon replaced by the beginning of true acclimatization, the physiological pathways followed as the sea level native responds to prolonged oxygen lack. There are many of these pathways, more subtle and less extreme than the struggles, each contributing a share to restoring cell oxygen toward normal. Over many years "acclimatization" becomes "adaptation"—similar responses inherited by the peoples who have lived for generations at altitudes as high as 5,100 meters (17,000 feet), the highest that humans can live permanently.

If you were designing these responses, you would want to pump more air, transport blood more efficiently, ease the passage of oxygen into cells, use fuels more efficiently, and discharge wastes more readily. You would want an easily available emergency supply of oxygen for extra effort, and you would plan the changes so that no part of the system wears out or breaks down prematurely. This is almost exactly how acclimatization works.

At sea level, arterial oxygen pressure is 110 torr and hemoglobin is 98 percent saturated; arterial carbon dioxide is about 40 torr, and the very close to pH 7.34. Any increase or decrease in breathing changes these numbers, sometimes considerably. By deliberately overbreathing we can maintain oxygen at a tolerable level, even as high as 7,500 meters (25,000 feet)—but only for a very short time before other imperatives intervene. The work of overbreathing is exhausting.

As we acclimatize over days and weeks, our natural responses change the numbers. On Everest's top the values are approximately: arterial oxygen 30 torr, saturation 45 percent, and carbon dioxide 12 torr, with a pH of 7.56. These are extreme values and only a few actual measurements have been made. How is it possible to survive such levels, especially if compounded by cold, exhaustion, dehydration, and other sapping stresses? The parameters measured even on lower mountains would be frightening if found at sea level.

Although overbreathing remains the primary, and most helpful, change in acclimatization, the heart does its share. In the first few days both heart rate and output increase, so more blood is pumped per minute. Then, as other changes evolve, the heart rate slows and output returns to normal and even (after ten days) falls slightly below normal. In general, the slower the pulse rate, the better acclimatized a person is considered to be. Interestingly, the ability of the heart to pump blood is not what limits humans at altitude. Even on the highest summit, the heart has reserves, though the muscles of respiration have little or none. Blood pressure increases somewhat in many people but not in all. After a few weeks it returns to normal in most people. Pulmonary artery blood pressure remains high throughout the stay at high altitude.

The more red blood cells and hemoglobin available, the greater the *capacity* of blood to carry oxygen, even when the decreased oxygen pressure decreases the oxygen *content*. Fluid re-enters the blood, and there soon follows a true increase in circulating hemoglobin as the blood-forming organs churn out more red blood cells. After only a few weeks at altitude, the oxygen carrying *capacity* is likely to be half again larger than at sea level. To a point this is helpful, but sometimes the response is too exuberant, and blood becomes so thick it actually impairs delivery of oxygen. This is the major problem in chronic mountain sickness

While these responses are maturing, ventilation remains high, sustaining oxygen pressure in the alveoli but lowering carbon dioxide. As discussed before, the two centers that control breathing are called on to respond in opposite directions—the one to increase breathing to prevent hypoxia, the other to decrease breathing to prevent excess loss of carbon dioxide (hypocapnia). How this conflict is resolved determines the success of acclimatization. Obviously a compromise is reached, and this is helped by a change in the blood that softens the drift toward alkalinity as the acidity from carbon dioxide diminishes. The major way this is accomplished is by loss of bicarbonate in urine—which is one reason why a good urinary output is so important. The increased hemoglobin also helps because it forms more buffers which also soften changes in blood pH.

We saw that some forms of hemoglobin acquire oxygen more readily and cling to it more tenaciously than others. This is most dramatic in the newborn where the fetal hemoglobin, ideally suited for life in the womb, changes to a transitional and then to an adult form. Fetal hemoglobin might be helpful at altitude, but it does not persist after infancy in humans. Other variants or mutants exist, but we have not adequately investigated those individuals with these different kinds of hemoglobin. A change in the hemoglobin molecule is not part of the acclimatization process, although its oxygen saturation curve is usually left-shifted.

It would seem desirable to improve the distribution of blood to many parts of the body by expanding the network of capillaries, thus bringing blood into closer contact with more cells. Does the body actually make new capillaries? Probably not. What does happen is that inactive capillaries are opened. Over time, both body fat and muscle decrease, so there are more functional capillaries per cross-section of tissue.

The cell of course is where the action is. Getting oxygen into each working cell is the "purpose" (if we can call it that) of breathing. It is the mitochondria in each cell that do the body's work. Are they changed during acclimatization? The evidence is unclear. It appears that after acclimatization, mitochondria may become slightly larger and be distributed closer to the perimeter of the cell, but they do not increase in number. Nor is it known whether or not they become more efficient.

Two more aspects of oxygen supply and demand should be mentioned. We say that oxygen is neither made nor stored in the body, but this is not exactly true: there are two functioning reservoirs from which oxygen can be drawn in time of need.

As already discussed, the best known is a myoglobin, found in muscle. The myoglobin oxygen saturation curve is left-shifted, which means that it easily acquires oxygen over a wide range of pressure, but discharges it reluctantly, at low pressure but in large volume. This neat arrangement means that when muscle is called on urgently to do extra work, an extra surge of oxygen is available. It would seem reasonable that myoglobin should increase during acclimatization, but the evidence is contradictory.

The second storage reservoir is in the blood returning through the large veins to the heart from all parts of the body. The oxygen content of this mixed venous blood indicates how much has been drawn by the cells and indirectly gives us an idea of the oxygen within them. It follows that the oxygen carried in this blood is a kind of store from which cells can draw when in need. In fact one study at extreme altitude found that acclimatized men drew down the oxygen in their mixed venous blood to a lower level than they were able to do even during maximum exertion at sea level.

This web of interrelated changes—and there are many more— make it possible for the sea level native to go very high if he gives his body time to adjust. Acclimatization takes many days or weeks depending on the altitude, and it cannot be rushed. Each person seems to have an individual pattern, and a fascinating question is whether once this pattern has been "learned," is it easier the next time. Anecdotally we have no doubt that it is.

The bottom line is that the net total of all of the changes of acclimatization make it possible for people to live and work with much less oxygen than they are accustomed to. And this applies to a limited extent to people who are short of oxygen at sea level due to some chronic illness.

What about the races that have lived for centuries in high places like the Tibetan plateau, the Andes, and Ethiopia? Have they followed the same paths of acclimatization? It is convenient to think that after generations at altitude, these people have adapted in the Darwinian sense, that evolution has chosen those changes which are most efficient and effective for life at altitude. As we study such natives we find that different races have developed slightly different strategies. Some have enlarged their chests to provide greater lung volume. Some have increased their hemoglobin. Some have developed more sensitive respiratory drives that are strongly responsive to oxygen lack, while others have blunted drives. Some races are short and stocky, others are tall and thin—though whether this is for oxygen economy is hard to tell.

Acclimatization, then, is an intricate network of changes in how we acquire, transport, and use oxygen, a process that takes time to develop, seems to be saved in memory, and after many generations produces lasting changes. Like mountain sickness the processes that produce it are not yet fully understood. Yet science is advancing rapidly, and it may not be long before future generations look back upon our gallant attempts at explanation with the same fondness that we today look back upon the efforts of Berti, Périer, Guericke, Bert, and so many others.

Finalé

Around 1540, Konrad Gesner's friend and fellow mountaineer climbed Mount Niesen, a small mountain near Interlaken in Switzerland. On the summit, carved in the rock were the words which can be translated "Love of mountains is best." This brief statement is of a piece with the more flowered poems and essays from ancient China, but expresses as much or more of the mountain spirit. It confirms also, that even few accounts survive, some of the ancients were moved by the some emotion which has led men and women onto high peaks for many centuries. In a sense is it not similar to the more intellectual love which leads us to explore the unknown in science? Is love of knowledge, a longing to explore, what leads us ever further toward understanding how our bodies function or fail? I believe so. Learning and teaching are noble human passions.

Perhaps we scientists may be likened to the travellers of whom James Elroy Flecker wrote:

We are the pilgrims master, we shall go
Always a little further; it may be
Beyond that last blue mountain barred with snow

INDEX

A

Acclimatization, description of, 63-68
Acosta, José de, 10
Acute mountain sickness (AMS), 45-47
A-hemoglobin, 32-33
Air
    composition of, 5-6
    necessity of, 3-4
Altitude illness
    acute mountain sickness, 45-47
    chronic mountain sickness, 57-58
    description of, 43
    factors affecting, 44
    high altitude cerebral edema, 54-57
    high altitude pulmonary edema,
        48-53
    high altitude retinal hemorrhage, 59
    preventing, 60-61
    sleep apnea, 58
    subacute mountain sickness, 58
    treatment for, 61-62
Alveolar hypoventilation, 57-58
Ammonium chloride, 61
Aristotle, 1, 25, 31

B

Barcroft, Joseph, 19, 27
Beeckman, Isaac, 1,11
Bernard, Claude, 37
Bert, Paul, 13, 31
Berti, Gaspar, 1
Blanchard, Jean Piérre, 12
Blood
    components of , 36-37
    oxygen in, 34-35
    role of, 23-27, 30-31
Borrichius, Olaus, 5
Boyle, Robert, 23, 4, 5
Brissey, Testu, 12
Buchner, Edward, 41
Buchner, Hans, 41
Byron, Lord, 7

C

Cavallo, Tioberias, 12
Cavendish, Henry, 12
Cells
    Krebs cycle, 41
    membrane transport, 39-40
    role of, 39
    role of red, 29-30

Cesalpino, Andrea, 26
Charles, J. -A. -C., 5, 12
Chauveau, Auguste, 27
Chronic mountain sickness (CMS), 57-58
Circulation, 23-27, 30-31
Citric acid cycle, 41
Colummbo, Renaldo, 26
Cournand, Andre, 27
Coxwell, Henry, 12-13

D
Dalton, John, 5
De Ville, Antoine, 10
Dexamethosone, 60-61
Diamox (acetazolamide), 60, 61
Diffusion, 17-18
Diuretics, 62

E
Empedocles, 8, 25, 31
Endorphins, 36
Erasistratus, 5
Erythropoietin, 30

F
Fetal hemoglobin, 32
FitzGerald, Edward, 43
Forssmann, WErner, 27

G
Galen, 16, 25, 31
Galien, Jseph, 12
Gamow Tent, 62
Gas laws, 5
Gay-Lussac, Joseph, 12
Gessner, Konrad, 9-10
Glaisher, James, 12-13
Guericke, Otto von, 1-2, 3
Gusmao, Laurenco de, 11

H
Hackett, Peter, 51
Haldane, John, 19
Hales, Stephen, 26-27
Harvey, William, 26
Hemoglobin
     oxyhemoglobin dissociation curve, 31-32

types of, 32-34
High altitude cerebral edema (HACE), 54-57
High altitude pulmonary edema (HAPE), 48-53
High altitude retinal hemorrhage (HARH), 59
Hobbes, Thomas, 8
Hooke, John, 31
Hooke, Robert, 3, 4
Hsien, Fa, 9
Hultgren, Herbert, 52
Hypoxia
     See also Altitude illness discovery of, 13-14

I
Ibn-al-Nafis, 26
Interstitial space, 20

J
Jourdannet, Denis, 13

K
Kobayashi, Toshio, 55
Krebs, Hans, 41
Krebs cycle, 41

L
Lana-Terzi, Francesco de, 12
Lavoisier, Antoine-Laurent, 5, 6
Leeuwenhoeck, Anthony van, 31
Leonardo da Vinci, 11, 25
Li Bai, 7
Liebig, Justus, 41
Lower, Richard, 31
Lymphocytes, 36

M
Malpighi of Pisa, 26
Marey, Jules, 27
Mayow, Joh, 3-4. 16
Membrane transport, 39-40
Methylene blue, 61
Meyer-Ahrens, Conrad, 13
Mitochondria, 41, 42
Monge's disease, 57
Montgolfier, Jacques-Etienne, 12
Montgolfier, Joseph-Michel, 12

Moss, Gerald, 52
Mountain sickness. See Altitude illness
Myoglobin, 33, 67
N
Nifedipine, 61
O
Oxygen
    in blood, 34-35
    capacity, 34, 66
    content, 34, 66
    responses to lack of, 41-42
Oxyhemoglobin dissocation curve,
    31-32
P
Pasteur, Louis, 41
Périer, Florin, 2
Periodic/Cheyne-Stokes respiration, 22
Peter II of Aragon, 9
Petrarch, 10
Philip of Macedon, 8
Pickwickian syndrome, 57
Pizzo, Chris, 64
Platelets, 36
Polo, Marco, 9
Priestley, William, 5, 6
Pulmonary Function Test (PFTs), 21
R
Ravenhill, Thomas, 43, 53
Respiration, 15-22
Richards, Dickinson, 27
Robert, A. J., 12
Robert, F. M., 12
Rozier, Pilatre de, 12
S
Scheele, Carl Wilhelm, 5
Schoene, Robert, 51
S-hemoglobin, 33-34
Servetus, Michael, 25-26
Simler, Josias, 10
Slepp apnea, 58
Smith, Albert, 10
Stadie, William, 19, 27
Stahl, Georg, 5-6
Starling, Ernest, 24

Subacute mountain sickness, 58
T
Torricelli, Evangellista, 1
Transfusions, 35
W
Whymper, Edward, 43
X
Xuandi, Emperor, 8
Z
Zang, Xuan, 9